Contents

About the author

Anita Houghton originally trained in medicine at the Middlesex Hospital, London, and specialised in public health medicine. After 12 years as a consultant, she moved into postgraduate medicine, helping junior doctors in difficulty, and instituting leadership and professional development seminars for registrars and new consultants. Over time she became increasingly interested in what motivated people at work, what made them happy and what made them excel. This led her to qualify as a professional and personal development coach. Using a combined approach of several disciplines, including psychological type and neurolinguistic programming, she has been helping people to improve their working lives for nearly ten years.

She is now advisor to the *British Medical Journal* working group on career development, an associate of the King's Fund, an organisation that provides management and personal development training to senior managers in the health service, and is a consultant on work-related problems, including bullying and harassment. She regularly writes articles on subjects related to personal and professional development.

In 2004, she set up The Working Lives Partnership, a coaching and consultancy service aimed at helping healthcare and other professionals to be happier and more productive at work — *see* www.workinglives.co.uk.

Part One

Getting started

1

Introduction

The healthcare professions are among the most demanding and most rewarding of all professions. Steeped in tradition, healthcare has been being provided for centuries, and under its auspices you will find the most conservative of practices, the most stereotypical of people, the most fundamental of human values. And yet within it you will also find the most cutting edge of technology and fastest pace of change, the greatest diversity of human beings, the toughest of choices. It is within these extremes that the healthcare professional has to find a home for their particular set of talents, characteristics and desires.

Work can be both our making and our undoing. A productive, successful and happy working life is a wonderful thing: inspiring, fulfilling and fun. An unhappy working life can not only ruin our working days, but has the ability to infect our whole lives with misery. Investing some time and effort in getting it right will therefore not only pay dividends in terms of short-term success and happiness at work, it will provide a framework for planning your entire working life, and have immeasurable positive effects on the rest of your life.

Many books on work and careers are centred around success, and the Western concept of success tends to be high status and much money. This book is different in that it is centred on fulfilment and happiness at work, and for two simple reasons:

- few of us want status and money at any price
- success follows happiness, as night follows day.

These are true for any profession, but in the case of healthcare it is especially unlikely that high status and earnings will be the primary motivation for entering its ranks. In most countries, healthcare professionals are not all that highly paid, either because healthcare is provided predominantly by the state, or because the professions are populated mainly by women. And even where money and status are more of a feature, most people attracted to healthcare are motivated at least in part by a wish to contribute to the society they live in. So while financial and societal prestige may well be a by-product of a successful career in healthcare, the primary aim of this book is to help the reader to find fulfilment and happiness in their work.

It is based on the following principles:

- Going inside to understand yourself is an essential first step towards a successful and happy career. Without understanding what makes you happy in life you are in a poor position to achieve it.
- When you know who you are and what makes you happy, you are empowered to review and plan your career with confidence.
- Once you realise that success and happiness are within your control in one area of your life, you've opened up the possibility that this could be applied to other parts of your life. The results are life changing.

Know and understand yourself

↓

Review your career/life in light of new knowledge

↓

Make necessary adjustments

↓

Notice results

Figure 1.1   The Know Yourself approach to career development.

If you work through this book I can guarantee that by the end of it two things will have happened: you will be in a much better position to plan and execute your future career, and you will feel a lot better than you do now. There will be times when you will wonder what some chapter or exercise has to do with your current situation, but if you want to get your career right, you need to do some groundwork, and that groundwork needs to be broad based.

Part One of this book is aimed at setting the scene, providing some background on typical career problems and their causes, and some strategies for getting in the right frame of mind for exploring yourself and your career.

Part Two covers the work each person needs to do in laying a strong foundation for career development. It asks what sort of person you are, why you work, what's important to you and what's important about you? It takes a close look at what you have to offer in the workplace and at what holds you back from offering it. In doing so it leads you to a greater understanding of the problems and dilemmas you are facing, or have faced in the past, and provides a framework for planning the future.

Armed with this new knowledge, Part Three takes you through a practical career development process which will ultimately lead to an action plan.

To complement this book, a workbook is available online at www.radcliffe-oxford.com/knowyourself.

What is *your* purpose in reading this book?

If you're an independent-minded sort of person you'll probably have only a passing interest in my purpose for you, and will be tempted to skip the section entitled 'How to use this book' in any book. You may want to work through the pages that follow methodically, or you may want to cut straight to one or two of the chapters that interest you; you may prefer to do it alone, or with a friend, or even a group of people. Whatever method you choose, though, I urge you to do one thing in preparation, and that is to clarify what you want from reading the book.

Clarify what you want from reading the book.

Take a few minutes to ask yourself 'What would I like to have for myself at the end of this book? What am I hoping to achieve?' It might be to:

- make a particular decision about a job or career move
- understand your current problems or dilemmas
- gain knowledge about your strengths
- generate a list of career options
- learn about career development in order to help someone else
- make a plan to improve your work–life balance
- increase your self-awareness
- something completely different from any of these.

When you have your desired outcome or outcomes, ask yourself 'If I had this by the end of the book, would I be pleased?' If you have any doubts, try adjusting your outcome until you're happy with it.

Once you're sure about what you want from the process, have a think about how you'll assess your success. What will you have to show for it? It may be a decision made, a plan drafted, a list generated, or it may be something less tangible, a new feeling of peace, an ability to move on from a past experience, or a sense of optimism about the future. When you know what it is you will have, ask yourself what it will be like when you have it. How will you feel exactly? What will you be seeing, thinking, hearing, experiencing? How will other people in your life be responding?

What are my outcomes for this process?

1

2

3

How will I know when I have these things?

1

2

3

What will it be like when I have these things? (What will I feel, think, see, hear?)

When you have your outcomes you are ready to begin. Work has the potential to bring great happiness. The aim of this book is to help you find that happiness.

2

Setting the scene

This chapter looks at the kinds of problems that people experience in their work, and the pressures that come to bear when we are choosing our careers. By the end you will be able to:

- set your own circumstances in a broader context
- understand more about the influences that have led you to where you are today.

Although we would all benefit from taking a measured, planned approach to career development, in practice, human beings tend to operate on the 'If it ain't broke, don't fix it' principle, having been provided with a nervous system that selectively excludes every shade of amber, but which leaps into a frenzy of activity when things go spectacularly wrong. So we amble along from day to day, responding to the pressures and opportunities of the here and now, enjoying what can be enjoyed and never taking the time to think through our working lives in any depth or breadth. Then one day it happens. It might be a nasty experience such as redundancy, divorce, death, illness, a restructuring or a difficult boss. It may be because a period of our lives has come to a natural end, as in leaving school or college, or coming to the end of a vocational training or contract. Or it may be a problem of a more internal kind – a sudden realisation that we're bored with what we're doing, an imperative to do something different, a reminder that life is marching by and if we're going to do anything exciting or worthwhile, we'd better get on with it.

You may be one of those rare people who seeks help well before problems take hold, but many people coming to a book such as this will be having some kind of crisis over their work. Something that is of immense help to anyone who is going through a work crisis is to know that they are not the only person who has ever had one. They are not the only person who has no idea what to do, has chosen the wrong career or job, has been made redundant, treated badly, had their competency questioned, been passed over for promotion, has subjugated their working lives to others, or has simply fallen out of love with their work.

It is impossible to go through life without things going wrong from time to time. These rough patches are part of life, and they have an important function. While governments and health services have tried for decades to get us to take more exercise, eat more healthily and give up smoking, healthcare workers know that there's only one thing that is guaranteed to make a person leave the house at six every morning in their jogging kit, eat fresh vegetables till they are coming out of their ears and sue the manufacturers of their favourite brand of cigarette instead of paying them. A nice big heart attack.

Work is the same. It's the easiest thing in the world to stay in a job you're not enjoying, or to go along with what someone else wants you to do. It's easy not to go for that promotion, that new job, that change in career. We like ease. To do something difficult takes a lot more commitment, a lot more energy and a whole load of courage. If you're low on these commodities, it takes a crisis.

A work-related crisis has the capacity to make you feel terrible. Work is a fundamental part of our existence, and a serious problem in our working lives can have all the charm of an earthquake. But while it's true that you can learn something of what you enjoy at work by doing nice things in nice jobs, you learn so much more when it all goes wrong. That's not simply because you need to understand what you don't like in order to understand what you do like (and there's much truth in that), but because it's only when things go seriously wrong that we wake up. Adversity has a way of standing up and shouting at us in a way that contentment does not.

So, if you're having a career crisis, welcome it with open arms. It's a great opportunity to take a good long look at your career and your life, and make a start towards getting it right. If you're not having a career crisis, then congratulations on taking avoiding action.

What kinds of career problem are there?

The most common kinds of career problem are those related to life stage, and just about everyone experiences indecision and confusion at one or more of life's stages. The first fertile period for career problems is during the latter years of school or university; and little surprise, as at this stage we are expected to decide what we would like to do with the rest of our lives. This is an extraordinary requirement of someone so young, and greatly hampered by a paucity of experience on the one hand and a surfeit of advice on the other.

The next period of life that has the ability to produce consternation comes a few years down the line, when you realise you've made a terrible mistake. Frantic with indecision in your late teens or early twenties, you finally plumped for something that seemed to be both possible for you and pleasing to those around you, but over the months and years it gradually dawns on you that you are about as suited to your choice of work as a wax saucepan is to cooking.

Then there's mid-life, which is thought to begin at any time between the ages of 35 and 50. You've been working quite happily at a job or career for some time, but you notice your enthusiasm for getting up in the morning is diminishing. Then one day you wake up and realise you'd rather be doing just about anything than going in to your current job.

One day you wake up and realise you'd rather be doing just about anything than going in to your current job.

And then there's the approach of retirement, with all its decisions about when to go, whether to wind down gradually, what you will do when you no longer have to work, and so on. And with people talking about the 'fourth age', the period of time after the three score years and ten that previous generations never expected to live beyond, the potential for career crises may be endless.

If life stage is the most common source of anguish when it comes to careers, the second must be change at work. You're in a job you enjoy, have colleagues you like, a supervisor or manager you respect and responsibilities that play to your strengths, and then bang! There's a restructuring, a merger, a new manager, a new directive, a new government, a new set of standards, a demand for different services, and everything changes. Suddenly there's a new boss who can't wait to put their stamp on everything. After years of doing a job carefully and competently, overnight you are no longer trusted, and a great swathe of documentation and auditing is introduced. Your nice, small hospital or practice is merged with another, much larger one, and you have to change the way you do things. You hear talk of redundancy or redeployment, and people have to apply for their own jobs; some see the writing on the wall and start leaving for greener pastures. Ways of working are changed and you find yourself with new tasks that are dull or difficult. All these have the ability to turn a thoroughly enjoyable job into a really grim one, and in a very short time. If there is a workplace anywhere that is immune to the modern propensity for continual change I'd like to know about it.

There are also more personal work crises that may sometimes be related to changes in the workplace. Few experiences precipitate a career crisis with the effectiveness and force of redundancy, for example, or being sacked, or taken through disciplinary procedures. Being bullied or harassed at work can be equally devastating, and with all these the crisis is deepened by the damaging effect these experiences inevitably have on your self-confidence and general wellbeing.

Another group of problems are those that arise from personal attributes. Perhaps you set out on a particular pathway and part of the way along you realise that your likelihood of progression is going to be seriously hampered by something you can do nothing about. Perhaps you find you are not clever enough, strong enough, thin enough, male enough, white enough or able-bodied enough. You've committed much time and commitment to a path, but it now appears blocked or impractical. What now?

Another source of potential difficulties are the changes a person may experience in the course of natural progression through the ranks of their profession. The job of a consultant, for example, is very different from that of a house officer in the same specialty, and junior doctors will sometimes look at what their consultant does and realise that it is not for them. Promotion to managerial roles may paradoxically mean an end to the kind of work that first drew a person to an area of work, for example taking a nurse away from looking after patients to managing teams and budgets.

And then there are the life events in our personal lives. There are the tough ones like divorce, death and ill health, although the nice ones, like marriage, starting a family and moving home, can be equally disruptive to a working life.

And finally there's you yourself. People change over time, often related to life stage and life events. Something we enjoyed at one stage in our lives may lose its appeal at another. A willingness to conform to corporate life may evolve into a desire to do your own thing. A drive to earn a lot of money may turn into a longing for time to pursue hobbies and interests. A commitment to caring for patients may become a commitment to caring for family, or a commitment to family may become an urge to do something for ourselves. Or we may quite simply want a change, for change's sake. Human beings are designed to need change. If you put a finger lightly on the back of your hand and leave it there, you will initially feel it, but after less than a minute the neurones stop firing and the sensation goes. A tiny movement and you feel it again. We need change for stimulation.

Sources of career problems and crises

- Life stage (leaving school/college, early working life, mid-life, retirement)
- Changes at work (mergers, redeployment, new bosses, promotion)
- Personal work problems (redundancy, sacking, performance problems, bullying)

- Life events (marriage, children, moving house, divorce, death, ill health)
- Personal attributes (age, gender, race, physical attributes, ability)
- Changes in you (interests, values, willingness to work for others)

How do people choose their careers?

A theme running through all these potential sources of uncertainty and anxiety is the whole business of career choice. While what you choose is not nearly as crucial as you might think, the question 'What shall I do?' is central to many a career emergency, and understanding the pressures and reasons that lead people to choose a particular direction can be helpful.

Sometimes, and quite wonderfully, people know exactly what they want to do, and they pursue it whether or not they have the right exam results, the right attributes or the support of their parents. With this kind of certainty they are more than likely to succeed. For many, though, the road ahead is less clear, and for these individuals there is no shortage of external pressures and expectations to push them this way and that.

Brains, culture and parents

Our first choices, and for an alarming number of us, our last, are made at school or university. Career choices at this stage tend to be based on exam results, cultural values, and the expectations of parents and significant others. Although career counselling at school and university has certainly improved in recent years, it still tends to be centred around academic achievement, and that is not always a good guide to what a person will find enjoyable and fulfilling.

Academic achievement is not always a good guide to what a person will find enjoyable and fulfilling.

Many people who find themselves on professional career pathways are multi-talented, high-achieving all-rounders, who could equally well have become a doctor or a lawyer, a manager or entrepreneur, a professional athlete or a musician. But some abilities are valued by our culture more than others, as are some professions, and that value is reflected not only in the prestige and status that is attached to these professions, but also in the financial rewards. The result is that the highly talented teenager who can play Bach fugues by heart on the piano and a mean game of tennis, has had major successes in school plays and received top grades for all their exams is much more likely to be channelled towards being a doctor than they are to becoming a musician, tennis player or actor. And there's a great deal of common sense in this, as you can always play the piano or tennis and act in plays as an amateur, but at the end of the day, most of us have a living to earn. The problem is that some people find themselves in professions which they are entirely able to do, as evidenced by a string of passed exams and promotions, but which they've never really enjoyed.

Ironically, less academically gifted individuals may stand a better chance of doing what they really love than their brainier counterparts. Take a young man who has never done very well at school and whose parents have regularly sighed 'What *will* become of him?' His self-esteem has been gradually eroded by a system that values academic prowess, and he knows he'll never make a lawyer or a doctor or a marine biologist. The major worry to his parents is less what he will do than whether he will do anything at all. Imagine their delight, therefore, when young Max suddenly announces that he would like to be a chef. Well yes, they say to themselves, he is a wonderful cook and perhaps he could make himself a living that way. Gradually, they realise, given that their son is not going to be the next Einstein, that being a chef has a certain ring to it that they could live with a great deal better than long-term drifting from one poorly paid job to another. So, no more quadratic equations and French verbs for Max. His parents enthusiastically support him in his endeavours, and at last he finds himself doing something he excels in and that he enjoys.

Imagine Naomi, though. The same age as Max, she has always been top of the class in everything academic. She sailed through primary school on a carpet of praise and prizes, straight into a highly academic, highly selective secondary school, which sends 20 pupils to Oxbridge every year, and turns out astrophysicists and cabinet ministers by the score. Her parents, who have already decided on her Cambridge college and have visions of her being a famous surgeon, are just thrilled with this child. Then one day Naomi announces that she wants to be ... a fashion designer. 'A FASHION DESIGNER!' comes the appalled response. 'OVER MY DEAD BODY!' And so it is that Naomi's private dreams become public, only to be crushed under the next truck.

Male or female?

Gender, of course, has an enormous part to play in career choice and development. Even though opportunities for women have increased immeasurably over the past 50 years, typical career pathways for men and women are still totally different. One of the reasons for this is that there are still many gender stereotypes in the workplace, and while some of this may be due to genuine differences between the sexes, much is due to tradition. Women traditionally nurture, and men traditionally lead, so in healthcare that has meant that women become nurses and therapists, while men become doctors and managers. Even in medicine, where more than 50% of medical students are now female, once qualified, women are much more likely to move into general practice and men are much more likely to become surgeons. There are still lamentably few men in the professions allied to medicine.

Typical career pathways for men and women are still totally different.

Another reason for gender differences in career choice and direction is that increased opportunities have not altered the biological facts of reproduction, and even where men wish to take an important role in child-rearing, women still bear the children and most want to play a significant role in their upbringing. While biology means a successful career may be seen more as a bonus than an expectation for women, the corollary is that men are under great pressure to succeed and be breadwinners. When couples have children, research shows that the women work fewer and fewer hours, while the men work more and more. Relationships where the woman earns more than the man have a higher failure rate than where the reverse is true, and if anybody gives up work in order to look after children, it's rarely the man.

In the professions where men predominate, people are expected to work long hours and are not expected to have a life that impinges on their work. In the UK, where for many years it has been possible for doctors with domestic commitments to train part time, it is still extremely rare for a man to take advantage of this, and men often complain of negative attitudes if they do. So men are under great pressure to conform with this long hours culture, whether they like it or not.

The result of all this is that while career pathways for men and women can look very similar in the early twenties, they look very different by the time they are in their thirties. Women will often start their careers very successfully, tail off while they have their families and have a resurgence of energy in their forties and fifties. Men will often work themselves to the bone, first to succeed in the eyes of the world and potential mates, and then to support their dependants, before grinding into a mid-life crisis in their forties or fifties. These different pathways can produce very different watersheds, and at very different stages in life.

Group norms

Traditions and norms within different subgroups of populations are responsible for a host of other influences on young people who are choosing their careers. Ethnic group, social class, family traditions – all exert influence and expectations on their members, whether it's to conform and stay within the group, or to sally forth and prove themselves in the world outside.

The good news

Despite all these pressures, many people do find their way into careers that fulfil, excite and satisfy them, and the reason is that specific career choice is not as crucial as you might think. This is largely because the things that people find important about their work tend to be general, rather than specific.

The things that people find important about their work tend to be general, rather than specific.

People often cite good colleagues as being an important source of job satisfaction, others cite intellectual stimulation, or a challenge, or helping people, or fun, or creativity, or a chance to work with their hands. These attributes are sufficiently general that they can be found in a host of careers. They are also facets that can vary within careers, and even between jobs that are more or less identical in content. A general practitioner, district nurse or manager, for example, would undoubtedly find practices where there were many colleagues who shared their values and interests, and practices where there were very few. So if you know what general qualities in work you're looking for, it is possible to generate large numbers of options where those qualities can be found. Indeed, you may only need to make very small changes in your current circumstances to find them.

Another factor that contributes to happiness at work is what you take to it, and that is totally under your control. There's a tendency in today's individualistic age to look at what a job or career is going to bring us, rather than what we're going to take to it. But these two things are inextricably linked. If you go to work with a spring in your step, a wish to contribute, and a kindly attitude towards your co-workers and clients, you have the potential to enjoy just about any job.

Finally, it's worth remembering that work is not the only part of your life. A characteristic of people having career crises is that work has assumed enormous proportions for them. Therefore the fact that they're unhappy in their jobs, or without a job, or don't know what to do, seems catastrophic and produces a sense of urgency to sort it all out that is not at all conducive to good career development. Having a well-balanced life not only gives you that spring in your step you need to make the best of work, but it reduces the impact of disaster in one particular part of it.

It's worth remembering that work is not the only part of your life.

3

Getting into the right state of mind

This chapter provides some first aid for the spirits. By the end you should have:

- a list of all you have achieved and are proud of
- dealt with and dispatched any disappointments
- a method for dealing with past traumas
- reviewed your current financial situation
- some strategies for being cheerful and positive.

Most people who seek help with their careers do so because they've hit the rocks in some way, therefore many who come to books such as this are in what you might call a suboptimal state of mind. The kinds of experience described in Chapter 1 have a tendency to produce an abundance of negative thoughts about yourself, other people, your prospects, your status, your financial situation, your ability, the world in general. Whatever you have decided about the source of your problems, it would be very unusual for someone to come through these thoughts and experiences with their confidence and self-esteem unscathed.

It is extraordinarily difficult to plan a career when your spirits are low. It saps your energy. It holds you back. It tells you that there's no point in trying such and such an idea because you'll only screw it up. Every option that looks attractive one minute looks unattainable the next. Don't be ridiculous, you tell yourself, I'm not capable of that. It is therefore extremely important that in any career-planning process you pay as much attention to your mental state as you do to your plans. Every chapter of this book is designed to increase your confidence while moving you forward, but this one provides a little first aid before you start the process.

What went well?

To feel low all you have to do is concentrate on what is wrong with you and your life, and to feel better all you have to do is concentrate on what is good. Reviewing our achievements is one of life's more enjoyable pursuits, yet we do it surprisingly rarely. How often do you sit down and tot up all your successes? How often do you run the associated pleasurable occasions through on your internal cinema screen? How often do you reward yourself for doing something well? How often do you *plan* to reward yourself, *in advance*? If you don't do these things you are missing out on a source of pleasure that is so very easy to experience. So much safer than bungee jumping. So much cheaper than a holiday. So much more available than sex. So much better for you than alcohol or marijuana.

I have a daughter of primary school age. She attends a fabulous school where achievements of every kind are praised and appreciated, not just the academic ones. Every Friday morning at assembly a number of certificates are given out. For some children it is for a piece of work they have done, for others it is for helping in a school activity, for another it may be for being kind to classmates, for another it may be for always being cheerful. Every child receives at least two certificates a term, and they value them.

What is so important about the certificate business is that it allows the praise to be tailored to the specific achievements or attributes of the individual child. It is always nice to be appreciated, but it is best when the praise is both specific and ties in with what we value in ourselves. Sometimes heads of departments or organisations give out general praise. Perhaps they send around a Christmas message telling the staff what a great year they've had, and thanking them for their contribution. Now if you live in a praise desert this might seem like a small but welcome puddle, but it will never substitute for appreciation for individual effort. We may have done well as an organisation, you think, but what have *I* done to contribute? Does the boss know? Does the boss even know I exist?

It often strikes me that adults are really just tall children. Our needs are exactly the same – we need to be valued, we need people to give us compliments, congratulate us on our achievements, motivate us and give us big hugs when things go wrong. The only real difference is that our culture has decided that adults should be self-reliant, self-motivated and not in need of hugs. The result is that most of us work in places where comments even approaching such praise are pretty thin on the ground. Bosses cannot be relied upon to lavish praise and encouragement. It is therefore extremely important to make sure you do it yourself. Regularly.

A little while ago a woman came to see me. A middle-grade manager in the health service, she had decided that it was time for a move and had asked me for help with an application for a job. She had told me she particularly wanted some help with confidence, and it turned out that she was having major difficulties with a colleague at work. From the start it was obvious she was low, and none of the talking we did about her application and what she needed to do to maximise her chances of getting it really lifted what was like a low mist hanging over her. A different strategy was required.

'What would you bring to this new job?' I asked her. She told me how much experience and knowledge she had, how she was good at getting on with people and getting disparate groups of people to work together. 'What sort of things have you done?' I asked her. And she described the projects she had organised, how she had facilitated others to develop their own ways of assessing how they were doing and developed systems to make improvements. 'And what else?' I asked her. And she told me more and more, so much more than when we first talked about why she was right for the job. 'And what did you do exactly that made all this happen?' I asked her. And she explained how she planned her projects, how she motivated people to become involved, how she supplied the resources people needed to complete their tasks. The more she told me, the more animated she became and the more I was able to see what drove this woman, how committed she was to her work and doing it well. By the time she'd finished I only wished I'd had a job to give her, there and then.

What she was doing in this process was going through all the things she was pleased with, her achievements and what is was about her that had made them possible. And I was encouraging her to be specific. Talking about her experience and ability to get on with people produced no spark at all, but when she remembered what those strengths had meant in practice, what a difference!

On another occasion I was consulted by a senior academic in a university department, successful to any onlooker, but unhappy. The source of his unhappiness, he told me, was that he wanted and needed to be a professor. He had two reasons for wanting to be a professor – he needed the credibility to attract research funding, and he wanted the status to feel good about himself, to boost his confidence. The root of the problem was that people younger, less experienced and less able than him had been given chairs, and this had sapped his confidence.

We set out on a process of finding out why he should have a professorial chair. As with my other client, he started off low key and uncertain, then became more positive and animated as he described all he had done, all he had achieved: his research, his book, his students, his specialist subject. Just giving him permission to blow his own trumpet for a while had turned him from a quiet and unhappy individual into a passionate and happy one. The interesting thing was that the next time I saw him he had done all the things we had worked out together for improving his chances of getting a chair, but had found in doing so, and in reviewing his achievements and what was important to him, that he had increased his confidence and sense of credibility to such an extent that he wasn't at all sure he needed or even wanted a chair any more.

It's quite possible to remember your triumphs without even a flicker of pleasure. To do that, you remember only the bottom line – I passed an exam, I got a job, I was promoted, I decided to study for something. Yeah, yeah, I remember that. You might think it unimportant now, you might have devalued it over the months or years, you might simply have forgotten how good it was. If you want to derive the most benefit from your achievements you must do more than that. You must remember where you were, what happened, who was there, how you felt, how others responded and what it meant to you. And then you must add in some new insights such as: How did I do that? What did I do that made this thing happen? What skills or qualities do I have that were important in this achievement? And so on.

It's also important to be very broad in your definition of achievement. Achievements may be big things like getting into college, qualifying as a professional, getting a great job. They can also be smaller things like getting to work on time, finishing a piece of work, having a good idea, learning a new procedure, doing something well, listening to a patient, helping a colleague, making a new member of staff feel welcome, being kind to someone when they made a mistake, praising someone, writing a document, handling a disagreement well, saying thank you, saying sorry. The more achievements you think of, the better you will understand what you do well and the better you will feel. Think especially about what you do that you might take for granted.

So now, list your achievements.

What have you achieved over the past two years that you are proud of? Take a LARGE piece of paper and make a list.

Now add any major achievements from longer ago.

For each one on the list, remind yourself:

- When and where was it?
- Who was around, and how did they respond to your achievement?
- How did you feel?
- What was good about it?

Then ask yourself:

- What did you do to make it happen?
- What specific skills and strengths do you have that made it possible?
- What did you do right that you would like to do again?

If in doubt about a particular achievement, ask yourself 'Is there anyone I know who finds this difficult?' The things you are best at are those you do unconsciously and with least effort. So if you are always in credit at the end of the month, remember that there are plenty of people who are not, and it may not be anything to do with how much they earn or how many dependants they have. If you always meet deadlines at work, remember the people who don't and ask yourself what you do that makes it possible. If you tend to be the one who remembers everyone's birthday, suggests social events and generally looks after people, remember how few people do that. Also think of the things you have done that have been difficult or frightening, but you've done anyway. In exploring your achievements, beware of the little voice that says 'That was nothing', 'Everybody does that don't they?', 'I didn't really do anything', 'It was mostly so-and-so', 'I could have done it better'.

Once you have your list, pick three or four achievements you are most proud of, and then pick three or four that you don't think are all that important. For each one, stop, close your eyes and remember it in specific detail. What happened, where were you, who was there, what did you do and how were you important in this situation? What did you do right that would be useful to do again, or that you would like to do more of in the future?

Things to be proud of ...

Getting a job, completing a project, getting a contract, passing an exam, learning a new skill, planning a project, recruiting new staff, moving on from a disappointment, learning from a failure, helping someone, being kind to someone, making a change, moving jobs, making a decision, making a speech, writing a letter, saying thank you, putting someone else first, tidying your office, solving a problem, saying I'm sorry, resolving a conflict, suggesting an outing, going to the gym at lunchtime, listening to someone's problems, speaking up at a meeting, being honest, sticking up for someone, going the extra mile.

What went less well?

Life is full of lessons. These lessons are repeated until you learn them.
From *Rules for Being Human*, John Seymour Associates NLP training manual.

Having looked at all that went well, it may seem a shame to bring ourselves down to earth with what didn't. Yet the truth is that however much we try to avoid thinking about our so-called failures, they are always lurking in the background and have a tendency to enter our minds just at the moment we least want them to. Perhaps you have had a bad relationship with a colleague, for example. It has damaged your confidence and though you have tried to put it out of your mind, it has a habit of popping up every time you consider befriending a colleague or asking them for help. Or maybe a patient complained about you or took legal action against you, and every time you find yourself in a similar situation you remember this. Maybe you once did a piece of work that was heavily criticised, and every time you start a new project there it is, hovering like a mosquito in your mind. No, the only way to deal with bad experiences is to face them head on, look at what went wrong and what you can learn from them, and then place them firmly in the nearest rubbish bin.

This is a time to have a good old clear out of all those damaging memories. What secret disappointments do you have lying around in the back of your mind? What are the negative pictures that appear just as you start a procedure or new piece of work? What are the experiences that hold you back from trying things, or that affect your performance when you do?

Examples of disappointments

Not getting a job, failing an exam, losing a friendship, a badly handled disagreement, a mistake at work, being complained about, being treated unkindly, treating someone else unkindly, ill health, a lost contract, a relationship split, losing money, continuing smoking, breaking New Year resolutions, not coping with a situation, failing to resolve a problem.

- How have you explained this disappointment to yourself?
- What was your contribution to this disappointment?
- What would you have liked to have done differently?
- What tips could you give yourself for the future?

For example, a young woman working happily and productively as an administrator had a change of boss. The boss didn't like her, complained about her work and when she failed to crumble, initiated disciplinary action against her. She knew that she had done nothing wrong, she joined a union and she prepared her defence. She won her case and the disciplinary action ceased without sanction or caution. This was a highly traumatic experience. Like any unprovoked act of aggression, it damaged this woman's confidence, not only in herself, but in the world at large. If it could happen once, it could happen again, the little voice says. Nevertheless, she took some valuable learning from the experience, and the more time that passed, the more she was able to learn.

These are the tips she gave herself as a result:

- People attack when they feel threatened, so take it as a compliment.
- You are your best defender. Make sure you prepare the evidence yourself, even if someone else is representing you.
- View monitoring following such an event as a form of protection for you.
- Whatever happens, remember, you can handle it.

An old proverb says 'What doesn't kill me, makes me stronger'. Reminding yourself of the ways in which you have grown stronger as the result of an experience is not just a positive way of dealing with it, it's a prerequisite for moving on.

I once had an unpleasant work experience myself. I was managing a research team and failing miserably. The members of the team had been in the organisation longer than I had and had their own way of doing things. They seemed to resent my position as manager and resisted all my suggestions and requests. They enjoyed working together and more or less froze me out. I was perplexed, as I had never had this experience before, and was successfully managing another team in the same department. What am I doing wrong? Why don't they like me? What can I do about it? I tried everything – spending more time with them, spending less time with them, organising social events, offering training, being nice, being firm, giving high performance ratings, giving average performance ratings, hinting at my concerns and talking directly about them. Nothing worked. Eventually I left the job, and although I was happy in my new work environment, I realised that my experience had taken its toll on my confidence. The main problem was that however much I pondered over the experience, I couldn't find anything positive to take from it. I racked my brains about what else I could have done, how I could have managed the problem better, all to no avail.

Some months later I was on a personal development course and I was telling one of the trainers about my difficulties in leaving this experience behind. A wise and kind man, he gave a smile of recognition. 'Ah yes,' he said, 'the trouble is that competent people are used to doing things well, and when they fail they keep on and on and on trying. I was once in that position myself,' he said, 'and in the end I realised that what I needed to learn was when to quit.' I realised even as he was speaking that this was the tip I needed for the future: Know when to quit. Some things just aren't going to work, and you need to recognise them. What would I have done differently if I'd had this tip then? I would have gone to the head of department, explained that for reasons I did not understand the chemistry in the team did not work, that it was damaging for everyone and that it would be best if I was put in charge of another team.

People stumble over the truth from time to time, but most pick themselves up as if nothing had happened.
Winston Churchill

If you look at a painful experience and just can't think of anything positive to take from it, ask yourself 'What did I do to maintain the problem?' You may not have created the problem, but if you were involved then you must have played your part in maintaining it. If you hadn't behaved the way you did, what else might you have been doing, and how might that have affected the situation?

When you have taken everything you can from your disappointments, run and put them in the nearest rubbish bin. They are of no further use to you.

Examples of tips

- Know when to quit
- Think before I speak
- Know when it is important to play the game
- Keep a sense of humour
- Listen to the other person's point of view
- Ask for help when I need it
- Treat holidays as an essential, not a luxury
- Look after my health
- Tackle important things first
- Open letters from the Inland Revenue

- Learn how to say no
- Walk round obstacles, not through them
- Put angry letters in a drawer for a few days

Dealing with trauma

Sometimes bad experiences are so upsetting that they come under the heading of trauma. In these cases, learning lessons may not be enough to leave them behind. Being singled out for aggressive or unkind treatment, for example, can leave a person in a state of deep anxiety, experiencing flash-backs, insomnia, nightmares and, as time goes on, maybe depression. It is not the place of a book like this to try and deal with such problems, but it is essential that they are dealt with and I offer one method of reducing the impact that the past has on the present.

One of the most distressing parts of trauma is our propensity to relive it. However much we try to occupy ourselves, think of other things, leave an experience behind, it stays resolutely in our thoughts, often in the form of memories of particular events. Perhaps you've been shouted at in front of colleagues, humiliated, criticised unfairly, disciplined, ostracised, ignored. You run the associated scenes through your mind again and again, and each time you experience the full horror. Sometimes they come during the day, sometimes they come, unbidden, at night. And every time they recur you experience the emotions all over again.

The idea of this next exercise is to reduce the impact of those memories by changing them. You may like to ask someone to take you through this, or do it alone.

Changing the past

First, select the traumatic event (or series of events) and identify a time before it started and a time when it was over. The story that unfolds between these two points will be your cine film.

Now think of a time when you felt great. Perhaps it was over a meal with a good friend, a family gathering, a work achievement, doing something creative. Take time to remember it in great detail, where were you, what were you doing, who was there, how you felt exactly, what you could hear, see, sense. Re-experience the good feeling as intensely as you can.

Now imagine a screen a little way from you and, keeping the good feeling, project the beginning of your film (before the traumatic event

Continued

---

began) onto the screen. You are now going to make a few changes to the film as you run it through:

- If your picture is in colour, imagine it now in black and white.
- Replace any sounds in the film with circus clown music, or any silly music you can think of.
- Now run the film through from beginning to end at the speed of a Charlie Chaplin film.
- When you reach the point when the trauma was over, stop, and then run the film backwards, still in black and white, at high speed and with the music.

If at any point you start to feel the trauma, stop and take a few moments to regain the positive feeling you started with. If the trauma still recurs, try placing the screen further away from you, making it smaller or imagining someone else watching it.

When you have finished the process, take a rest and then think of the events again. See if there are any differences in the way you feel. If not, try again, either now or on another day. This technique really does work in taking the emotions out of a memory.

Getting help

If you are severely distressed you should get help, and there is no shame in doing so. Friends and family are invaluable at these times, of course, but sometimes you need to talk to a professional who is totally uninvolved. Many organisations provide counselling support for their employees, and this is a time to take advantage of it. Your general practitioner is another source of help, and they should be able to assess your stress levels and suggest a course of action, whether it is taking time off work, being referred to a counsellor or a short-term pharmacological solution.

You may want to access coaching or counselling independently, and if you do, you need to think about how to find the right person. In the UK there are registers of qualified counsellors/coaches maintained by the British Association of Counselling Services (BACS) and by the Association of Neurolinguistic Programming (ANLP), both accessible via the Internet. To improve the chances of finding the right person for you, ask around for personal recommendations from people you like and trust. When you check out a particular coach or counsellor, find out the areas in which they specialise, for example work-related problems, relationship problems, phobias and so on, and whether they deal with deep or relatively superficial problems. When you've found someone you wish to approach, speak to them on the telephone first and ask about their approach to therapy, and consider if it will suit you. Some people are looking for quick, effective ways of moving forward, as in the 'changing the past' technique described above. Others are more interested in examining root causes of their problems, perhaps as far back as their childhood, and are looking for sustained psychotherapy over a period of time. Be clear about your needs and how the therapist plans to meet them.

Money

The main thing that stops people from leaving jobs they hate is the money. To walk away from a steady income to uncertainty and potential poverty is a very hard thing to do. We all have a lifestyle to maintain, but if you have dependants it is even harder because not only are you plunging yourself into a financially challenged situation, you are doing the same to them.

If money is a major issue, it's worth doing an inventory of what you need to survive, compared to what you have. If there is a shortfall, you are at risk of making hasty decisions about your career in order to close the gap as quickly as possible, and you need to have a think about how you could manage while you make your plans. Could you reduce your living expenses for a while? Do you have savings you could draw on? Are there people in your life who could help you out in the short term? Could you take a temporary job, or provide services as a freelance for a while? Are you entitled to benefits?

It's helpful to remember that any stop in the flow of money into your life is only going to be temporary. Healthcare professionals are of great value all over the world, so the chances of being involuntarily unemployed for any period are very low. Not only that, but you are taking active steps to sort out your career, so it is only a matter of time before you have a job you enjoy.

Taking positive action to raise your spirits

We are a cause-and-effect society, and when we're unhappy or otherwise distressed, we like to look for a cause and then treat it. The frequent assumption is that the cause is outside ourselves, and if we can only find it, we can either eliminate it or leave it. But it's not as simple as that. Happiness is a

---

Survival income

	Monthly £	Could reduce? Y/N
Rent/mortgage		
Local taxes/community charge		
Water		
Electricity		
Gas		
Telephone/mobile		
Clothing		
Television licence/subscriptions		
Hire charges (TV/video)		
Food/housekeeping		
Insurance		
Car/motorbike		
Interest/repayment on loans		
Entertainment/holidays		
Subscriptions (professional, clubs)		
Children's expenditure/fees		
Total outgoings:		
Income from partner/family:		
Other income:		
Savings:		

---

habit, not an effect, and its secret lies in what we are, how we think and what we do, rather than what happens to us.

If there is one thing that has changed my life more than anything else in recent years, it is the discovery that I have choice over how I feel. There are many different tricks, and everyone will have their favourite. Here are a few.

Do nice things

Make a list of things you enjoy. Who or what are the people, places, activities and experiences that make you feel good? Imagine doing some of these, take a bit of time to experience the pleasure of doing them, and get out your diary and schedule a few.

Be creative

When was the last time you drew a picture, decorated a room, wrote something, made something, grew something, cooked a nice meal? Do something creative.

Be active

What kinds of exercise do you enjoy? Do you like walking or running in the open air? Do you like working out at the gym? Do you like tennis, golf, football, cricket, basketball? Do you enjoy gardening? Or do you like the idea of more gentle or meditative activity such as yoga, Pilates or t'ai chi? Plan some regular activity that you enjoy.

Write down your thoughts

This can be very cathartic at first and release a host of pleasant, creative juices if you do it regularly. It is best done first thing every morning; take a pen or pencil and some sheets of paper, and just write whatever comes. Don't stop, don't reflect, just pour the flow from your brain straight onto the paper for about ten minutes. Don't worry if it's complete gibberish!

Keep your thoughts positive

It's more or less impossible to stop thinking. You might achieve it for brief periods of time if you meditate regularly, but thoughts always creep back in time. The challenge is to exert some control over their content. First you need to become aware of your patterns of thought. What do you think about when you first wake up, during the day, when you are in bed at night? If you are unhappy or stressed, the chances are that you devote much time to thinking about people or events or situations that produce negative emotions.

Try paying some objective attention to your thoughts. Become curious as to what goes on in your head, and notice the effect your thoughts have on the way you feel. When you have identified the thoughts that make you feel good and the thoughts that make you feel bad, make a conscious effort to spend more time on positive thoughts and let negative thoughts float out of your head as you become aware of them.

Generate positive feelings

Have a look at your list of what you enjoy, select one of the people, activities, places or experiences that you really love, and imagine it in its full glory. If it's a person you love, imagine being with that person and experience the feelings you have for them. Notice where in your body that feeling starts, and imagine that it's a warm fluid that spreads gradually around your body, filling your head, your limbs, your chest and abdomen. If you like, give the fluid a colour and imagine it reaching into the very tips of your fingers and toes, and when all your body is full of this warm fluid, imagine it circulating around you, up and down your spinal cord, around your brain, back into your chest and limbs.

The wonderful thing about this technique (adapted from *The Endorphin Effect*, by William Bloom) is that you can do it anywhere, any time: when you wake in the morning, or go to bed at night; as you walk down the street; sit at your desk; absolutely anywhere. Do this at least once a day for ten minutes and your mood will lighten, and not only will you be able to generate good feelings at will, but in time they will come upon you by their own volition.

What is your situation right now?

Finally, as you sit and read this book, ask yourself 'Is my life at risk?' A strange question, you may think, but it is posed to make the point that unless your life is at risk, at this very moment, you have no cause to panic. Anxiety is almost entirely produced by thoughts of what might happen and it deprives important tasks of valuable energy.

Take a few minutes to think about what is currently good about your life. Is your health good? Are you physically safe? Do you have a roof over your head? Do you have family and friends? Do you have enough to eat? Is there any money at all in your bank account? Do you have an income, from earning or some other source? Did the sun come up this morning?

Is there any reason for you to be anxious or unhappy at this very moment? If not, well isn't that nice?

Part Two
The groundwork

4

Why do we work? Money

This chapter looks at the main driver for work — money. By the end of it you should have a better understanding of:

- the importance of money in your life
- how you spend money
- what you believe to be 'sufficient'
- the balance between money and happiness that you have struck in your life, and what you might be prepared to trade.

Let's not beat about the bush here — the main reason we go out to work is for money. There are certain things we do for nothing in life — loving, eating, drinking, bathing, sleeping, having children, making a home, having fun — but going out to work is not one of them. Even people who claim that their work is their hobby expect to be paid. That's simply because most of us have to earn a living.

Many years ago I did a correspondence course in journalism and I remember a question that was posed in the first module: Why do you want to write? Apparently people answered this in a variety of ways: I've always enjoyed writing, people tell me I write a good letter, I'm interested in words, I want to voice my ideas and thoughts, I'd like to help people with my writing, and so on. 'All wrong!' said the tutor, 'none of these are a good reason to write. You must want to write first and foremost because you want to earn money from it.' Of course that doesn't have to be the reason you want to write, but what it was trying to say was that this was the assumed purpose of the course. The course was not to help you write — if you don't want to sell your writing you can write whatever you like, however you like, as misspelt and inelegant and misinformed and boring and annoying and inappropriate and irrelevant and ungrammatical as you like. If you want to sell it though, you need to learn how.

Therefore, prosaic though it may seem for a book which is aimed at discovering the 'real you', it is important to remember at all times that careers are first and foremost about earning. If you are in the unusual position of not having to earn a living, you may be more interested in the less profitable aspects of work, but for the majority who have a living to earn, there are a number of things to remember when it comes to planning a career.

First, if you want to earn a living at something you have to learn how to do it, and you must become sufficiently proficient that people are prepared to let you loose in their workplace and pay you for it.

Second, it's important to find something you enjoy doing and in a place you find congenial; partly because you are going to be spending a large proportion of your waking hours doing it and also because if you don't like it, it's not easy to decide one day that you will no longer go in. People don't pay you if you do that, and if you don't get paid neither do your bills.

Third, if you work for a living you make a deal with a person or an organisation that in return for your time and skills, they will give you money. At any time, that person or organisation may decide for a variety of reasons that they no longer wish to continue with the deal. Working for your living is therefore inherently insecure, and it's important that you have skills that can be used in more than one setting.

Finally, it is important to realise that when you work for someone the rules are largely set by that person. That again is the deal. So while the aim of this book is to guide you towards work that is both meaningful and enjoyable, a mental attitude that views employment as a game that you have chosen to play is useful. If you don't like the rules, or choose to go against them, then you need to be prepared for the consequences.

The extent to which you are affected by these factors will vary depending on whether you are employed or self-employed, but everyone who needs to earn a living depends on someone else to give them money for their services or products. The only important differences between employment and self-employment are degrees of security and autonomy.

The assumption, then, in career development is that the need to earn a living is implicit. People may say that money is not important to them, but unless they have independent means that can never be true – what they mean is that money is important, but they're prepared to trade in some money for other things.

Attitudes to money

Money is a source of conflicting emotions for most of us. There is something a little dirty about money. In Europe, we live in a culture where if you have it, it's not nice to flaunt it. Be casual about it. Be subtle about it. Preferably inherit it. Hence the expression 'nouveau riche'. Yet we have national lotteries and football pools and betting shops and bingo, and all manner of activities aimed at getting people to risk what little they have for a chance of having a lot more. And they do it in their millions, every day, all over the world.

For we all know that money is great. We love having it. We love what we can do with it. We love the freedom it buys us, the lack of worry, the luxuries, the gifts, the holidays, the houses. Let's give ourselves a break and admit, just quietly, but with glee, that we love it. We would like more of it. If someone arrived with a large cheque from the estate of some distant relative, we would accept it, wouldn't we? We might consider carefully if we wanted to change our lives, we might wonder what problems it might pose and what good causes we could support with it, but on the whole we'd take it wouldn't we?

I've been miserable and poor, and I've been miserable and rich. Miserable and rich is better.
An American actress

The question then arises as to relative value. How much do we *value* money as compared to other things in our lives? How much do we *need* money as compared to other needs in our lives? How much do we *desire* money as compared to other desires in our lives? What do we want from money, and what does it get for us?

The answer to these questions varies considerably from person to person, and depends, of course, on circumstances. If you are poor and hungry and without shelter, money is a necessity simply for survival. For many, perhaps most of us, money is about security. It buys us not only the necessities and comforts of life, but peace of mind. Our entire lifestyle depends on how much money we earn – our home, our food, our car, our mobile phone, our holidays, our leisure. The trouble is, it's difficult to enjoy a lifestyle if you don't know if you're going to have it tomorrow, or next month, or next year. Some people manage uncertainty in their lives better than others, but there is little doubt that for most people a real threat of unemployment, or serious loss of money for some other reason, causes enormous anxiety and stress. An entire industry both depends on this anxiety and feeds it. We pay into pension schemes for financial security in our old age, insurance schemes to insure our cars, our houses, our health, our possessions, our children's education, our fitness to work. We even insure our insurances, for heaven's sake! Suffice to say that financial security is important to most of us.

Tied up with security is the ability that money gives us to look after our dependants, and to provide the standard of living we would like them to have. It allows us to fulfil what we see as our duties in life, and to fulfil our duty is an important source of self-esteem. Also good for our self-esteem, we value the status and associated confidence that money gives us. Why else would people spend so much of their hard-earned income on the outward signs of success? Why would they spend more than they need to just to buy a particular brand? Why would they be prepared to go into serious debt to buy something they could easily do without? And the sad irony is that the less money you have, the more important it becomes to demonstrate to the world that you can afford to buy these things.

> *Many people spend money they haven't got, to buy things they don't want, to impress people they don't like.*
> Laurence Boldt

Even if you believe yourself to be immune to the lure of unnecessary possessions, everyone relies on money to a degree for their status and confidence. Because people tend to mix with others of similar financial means, the need for money to maintain social standing is not always obvious, but find yourself among people with a great deal more money than you and it's hard not to feel uncomfortable. You may have enough self-esteem to be undaunted by such differences, but even so, mixing with these people on a regular basis wouldn't be easy. If your idea of a night out is a few beers and chicken in a basket down at the local pub, for example, finding yourself among people who frequent gastronomic restaurants would be awkward to say the least. And mixing with people of considerably less means can be just as uncomfortable. So even though we may not always be aware of it, our financial status does buy us confidence and ease within our social group.

Independence is also something many of us value about money. A non-working woman married to a man with a good job may derive much from him in the way of confidence, status and standard of living, but if he dies, or runs off with his secretary, where does that leave her? Similarly, having an unearned income arising from family wealth may give a person substantial material means, but again there is a price to be paid. I once overheard such a person talking on the telephone to his father. Standing to inherit a substantial fortune on his father's death, he was being asked (in front of a number of guests) to explain why it was that his son had made a number of spelling mistakes in a recent letter, despite the large amount that his grandfather was spending on his education. To witness such a humiliating conversation was all the assembled company needed to convert their envy of his life of easy indolence into a renewed enthusiasm and gratitude for work. Having access to someone else's money may give us status, confidence and a degree of financial security, but earning your own money gives you control over that access.

Money can also bring freedom – freedom to purchase, freedom of movement, freedom of time. If you have enough, it also buys you freedom from worry about money, and there are few greater luxuries than that. And although we undoubtedly spend money on items that we neither need nor really want, money also buys commodities we do value and the means to access what's important to us. If you wish to be a musician, for example, money buys instruments, tuition, music, recording equipment. If you enjoy photography, money will buy you a good camera. If you like foreign travel, you need money for transport, accommodation and sight seeing. Money can buy you an education for yourself or your children, and is more or less essential for being able to choose where you live, what you do with your holidays and how you spend your leisure time.

Last but not least, money can bring fun. Having luxurious possessions and going on expensive holidays can be very enjoyable, as can giving a large amount of money to a good cause or to people you like, or even to people you don't know just to see their reaction. When we've fulfilled our duties, it allows us to be generous with what is left over, and there are few greater pleasures in life than to give. Throwing parties, expensive amusements, eating out, designer clothing, jewellery, fast cars, yachts, planes, second and third homes ... there's no end to what you can spend money on if you have it. Manufacturers and advertisers make sure of that.

That people are so extraordinarily creative in the ways they find to increase their income tells us a huge amount about the power of these drives for money and what it can buy. Earning is, of course, one way, and the method this book is devoted to, but the gap between what people want and what they think they are capable of earning can sometimes look as wide and as deep as the Pacific Ocean. So people dream of legitimate 'quick buck' methods: writing a best seller, inventing something, discovering something, becoming famous. Then there's marrying money, winning money, inheriting it. Increasingly, people are turning to litigation as a way of boosting their means. And then, of course, there's crime. Crime is a direct result of people wanting what they don't feel empowered to get through legal means.

What does money mean to you?

Take a bit of time to think through how money is important to you, and what drives you most in the quest for money. Anyone who studies medicine, for example, knows that part of the package is a relatively secure and above-average salary, and however altruistic the motivation for studying medicine, money will be at least part of the attraction. Being a student for five or six years is good preparation for understanding the importance of money in your life. If you are still a student and do not have rich parents who send you fat cheques every so often, what have you found to be the ups and downs of relative poverty? What are you most looking forward to about having a decent income? What might be the downsides? If you have a good salary, think of what you have access to that others do not, and imagine what it would be like without those assets. Sometimes people have money and then lose it, or decide to walk away from it. Again, the contrast will give special insights into the advantages and disadvantages of money, and the freedoms and obligations that go with it.

In the days we had nothing we had fun.
Harvey Andrews, folk singer

When you've thought through what is important to you about money, write it down. Then look at your list and ask yourself, if you could have all but one of these benefits in your life, which would you be prepared to lose? When you have done this once, repeat this process until you have prioritised your list.

Make a list of what is important to you about money

1
2
3
4
5
6

Now place the above in order of priority

1
2
3
4
5
6

When you've worked through the benefits, have a think about the price you pay for having money. What are the downsides of having money, depending on it, being responsible for it? What have you subjugated in your life in order to have it? The man mentioned earlier who lived on family wealth had paid the price of independence and dignity. While his lifestyle relied on a steady flow of cash from an irascible and demanding parent, he would have to put up with being called to account for the money he spent. He had also paid with his potential, because while money would have allowed him freedom to pursue whatever occupation he wished, in practice the lack of financial imperative had led him to do very little.

For the majority who work for their living, or depend on someone who does, the price to be paid for money is rather different. If we want to preserve a lifestyle we need to do whatever it takes to ensure that sufficient funds keep finding their way into our pockets or bank accounts. We may pay for this with our time, subjugating leisure, or family, or even health to the imperative to earn not only enough for now, but more in the future. We may pay with our freedom, staying in a relationship, for example, more because we are tied to the income than because we are tied to the person; staying in a job more because we like the salary than because we like the work. We may pay in terms of responsibility. Having money and possessions entails organisation, vigilance, planning, maintaining, administrating, investing, worry. Relying on money also tends to involve playing the game – deferring to people we don't wish to defer to, obeying rules we disagree with, engaging in activities we would rather not, belonging to groups we feel alienated from.

What is sufficient?

> *If you follow the God of More, you never win. Because there always is more.*
> Charles Handy in *The Hungry Spirit*.

It's likely that human beings have always faced the choices of security or freedom, caution or adventure, prudence or extravagance, but perhaps it is the combination of the all-pervasive media in Western society and a decreasing reliance on things spiritual for our sustenance that has led us to what must be an unprecedented pressure to have money. These days, with mass advertising, you don't have to mix with people who have more money than you to know that they exist and to feel dissatisfied or inferior in some way. Designed at undermining the individual while offering material solutions, advertising bombards us with images of beautiful, successful and wealthy people and their expensive accessories. Will you ever be able to hold your head up if you don't have the sort of income that is needed to buy these things?, is the wordless message.

Are you ashamed of your mobile phone?
From a UK television advertisement for a mobile phone

Unless you're clear about what money means to you and how much you are happy to settle for, you risk being jostled forever by the endless stream of advertisers whose aim it is to play on those feelings of insecurity. The question arises, therefore, what is sufficient? The Greek philosopher Epicurus, famed for his pursuit of the good life, believed people needed very little money in order to be happy. Happiness, he claimed, increases with the acquisition of money while you're moving from want to sufficiency, but as soon as you reach sufficiency the relationship tails off (*see* Alain de Botton, *Consolations of Philosophy*). In fact, happiness may actually decrease, Epicureans have since said, because having more money takes you into the world of consumerism, with not only the constant desire for more, but the loss of freedom that goes with being dependent on earning money. They have also pointed out that inherent in a life of consumerism is substituting the satisfaction of our real needs with material possessions. Epicurus' concept of sufficiency was to have enough for the bare essentials of life – food, clothing and shelter. His other ingredients for happiness were freedom, friends and thought.

It might be tempting to think that things were different in the Athens of 300BC, and that it was easier to live on the bare essentials then than it would be now. In fact, what Epicurus had to say in his philosophy makes it clear that the choices between luxury and simple living were just as potent then as they are now. While some sociologists will tell you that poverty is an absolute measure, that it exists when someone does not have sufficient means to have food, shelter and clothing, most are of the opinion that poverty is relative. So if you live in a country where the majority of people have a television, a washing machine, a telephone and a car, and you have none of these things, that would be termed poverty. In the late 1990s, a British cabinet minister stated that people were 'disadvantaged' if they did not have access to the Internet, something that nobody had even heard of only a few years before. In the Western world, therefore, if you decided to live on the bare essentials you would be taking yourself, and any dependants you may have, into relative poverty.

However, there are degrees between riches and poverty, and increasing numbers of people in our society are deciding to draw the line of sufficiency rather lower than the advertisers would like. So many are deciding they would like to trade in some of their money for a more enjoyable lifestyle that there is now a name for it — down-shifting. That a significant proportion take themselves off into the countryside, either in their own country or abroad, tells us not simply that they would like a rural existence as part of their lifestyle change, but that living on very little may be easier in the middle of nowhere than in the town, where the pressures to spend are greater and differences more visible.

Money and career choice

Your desire for material possessions and your ability to decide what is enough can have a huge bearing on your choice of career. If you are looking at the modern world of consumerism and wondering how on earth you are going to achieve and maintain a standard of living that includes access to most of what it offers, there are many careers you will have to scrub before you even start to consider your options. That's not to say that earning a great deal and pursuing a career you will enjoy are mutually exclusive, but simply that if you wish to earn a great deal, the pool of careers from which you can choose will be smaller.

I recently met some students in their final year at Oxford University and they had some interesting stories to tell. Manufacturers know that the bright young things who make their way into prestigious universities are likely to be the trendsetters of the future, and they expend considerable effort and money in recruiting these people to their cause. It's not uncommon, for example, for the best-looking, brightest students to be paid for wearing certain labels of clothing, for drinking certain alcoholic beverages and for smoking certain brands of cigarette.

Potential employers also understand that the cream of national intelligentsia are at these universities, and final-year students find their pigeon holes crammed with brochures from large city firms inviting them to join their graduate programmes and offering extraordinarily high starting salaries. When you are an impoverished student with a large debt to repay, how difficult must it be to push these temptations aside and go for less lucrative careers?

Inevitably, the decisions that most of us come to are a balance of many, often conflicting, factors. We decide what we would like to do, we assess what we are capable of, we look at a lifestyle we would wish to emulate and we weigh up our options. If we find ourselves capable of pursuing a career we think we'd enjoy and that will produce sufficient financial rewards to achieve or maintain our desired standard of living then the decision is easy. If, on the other hand, these factors fail to line themselves up in a neat row, or if one or more or them changes along the way, then difficult choices have to be made. It is easier to make these choices if you have a clear idea of what money means to you and a good understanding of the things it buys that genuinely enhance your life and those that you frankly would not miss.

A personal stock-take

Have a think about how you spend your money now. If you're not someone who normally monitors your expenditure, hazard a guess as to the proportion of your income you spend on your home, food, leisure, clothes and so on. When you've done that dig out your bank statements for the past few months and see if you were right. Add it all up, and for each main category of expenditure ask yourself: What does this bring me in life? What is my underlying motive for spending money in this way? How would my life change if I stopped spending money on this?

Take clothing, for example. The amount we spend is usually way over what we need to keep warm and avoid being picked up by the police for indecent exposure. Deborah, a consultant rheumatologist in her late thirties, told me she had never been extravagant in buying clothes and was surprised to find from her bank statements that she did spend a modest amount most months. When I asked her what this expenditure brought her in life she came up with fun – she enjoyed buying and having new clothes – and credibility – many patients still expected their consultant to be male, so she felt the need to look smart and professional. When I asked her what would happen if she didn't buy any new clothes for two years she was surprised to find that her first instinct was 'not very much'. She had a wardrobe, she told me, of perfectly good clothes. We agreed that fashion is so catholic these days that it's difficult to look seriously dated, and large swings in style tend to be aimed at the very young. She then realised that one effect would be that she would value what she had more, take more care of her clothes and review her wardrobe from time to time to check what was there. In the end she began wondering if maybe she wouldn't buy any clothes for a couple of years.

Work through all your areas of expenditure, each time exploring the benefits of spending money and the consequences of not. Once you've finalised your list of spending categories and have some clarity about what benefits these things bring you in life, ask yourself what this means in terms of what is important to you (*see* Chapter 7). To what extent does your expenditure reflect your values? Which expenditures are essential to satisfy what is important to you? Which expenditures are unnecessary?

How do you think you spend most of your money?

Check through your bank statement or cheque book for the last few months and add up how much you spend on each main category (e.g. house, clothes, holidays, travel, food, etc.). For each one, ask yourself 'What does this get for me?'

Category of expenditure   Average monthly spend   This gets for me?

How would your life change if you stopped, or substantially reduced, expenditure on each of these categories?

The balance between money and meaning

Most of us dream about having a substantial unearned income. This is never more appealing than when you are disenchanted with your work. At times of stress, unhappiness or burnout, winning the lottery can look like the arrival of the cavalry in a siege. Even when happy at work, most people will pass pleasant hours imagining they have a vast amount of money. For many of us the fantasy is accompanied by the deafening sound of shackles falling – no more worrying about paying the bills, no more scrimping and saving, no more choosing the cheapest items off the menu, no more bowing and scraping to the boss, no more being shouted at by ungrateful patients, no more being condescended to by small officials in smart places. Then come all the things we can buy that we have never been able to afford – the houses, the cars, the accessories. Then come all the things we can do, all the places we can go, the presents we can give and the parties we can throw.

Funnily enough, most fantasies tend to stop around there, rarely proceeding beyond the first few weeks. But what would it really be like if you had several million pounds in the bank? How would you feel if you knew you never had to earn again? How would you feel in relation to other people? Would you really give up working, and if so, how would you spend your time? I posed these questions to Julian, a clinical psychologist, and the first thing he noticed was a feeling of confidence and ease, followed swiftly by a sense of freedom. This was a revelation in itself, as he had never realised that having independent means would make him feel so confident in relation to other people. Then he wondered if he would give up his job and devote himself to writing a book and perhaps seeing a few private patients. For a few minutes this seemed an attractive prospect and a welcome relief from the pressure and human misery to be found in the health service, but then he realised he would miss his colleagues, the structure of going in to work and the feeling of doing a worthwhile job. Next he thought he could replace all that by getting involved in local community groups, which would give him companionship and a sense of purpose. He would form a network of other writers perhaps, strike up friendships with local people, play golf, plan a routine for himself. He became so carried away that in the end I had to remind him gently that he didn't have a private income.

Have a play around with these thoughts and questions. Notice the way you feel as you toss around the different scenarios. If something feels really good, before you discard it as a pipe dream, ask yourself if it really might be possible. There are plenty of people who have an unearned income, after all. But also recognise what you might lose if you had no need to work, for these are the clues as to what is important to you about work. The purpose of asking ourselves these questions is to tease out what is important to us about money, and in the context of work, where does the importance of money begin and end? As we have explored earlier, for all of us who have to earn, money buys the necessities in life, for ourselves and our dependants. After that it buys us what we value in life, and after that it buys us luxuries – possessions and experiences that are not essential but are fun. Everything else we gain at work we could put under the heading 'meaning', qualities in our lives that money can't buy.

While the ideal job would be rewarded with a salary that allowed you to live the lifestyle of your choice and provide you with all the qualities you would wish from your work, in practice we usually have to balance these elements. A highly paid job may include more responsibility than you are comfortable with, for example, or longer hours than you would wish. The questions you may ask yourself are: Does the pay compensate for having very little life outside work? For doing an inherently stressful job? For spending much of the day travelling? Are you compromising anything you value in order to have this highly paid job?

On the other hand, a very rewarding job may not pay well. Jobs such as nursing and working for charities are often highly rewarding, but poorly paid compared to other professions. If you're in this position, the questions you may ask yourself are: Do the rewards of the job compensate for having so little money? For being unable to care for your dependants in the way you would like? For living in a place you don't like, because you can't afford to buy anything better?

These difficult equations can face people at any stage of life, and as with most things, our priorities can change with time. Someone who follows their heart into a low-paid job may tire of poverty as time goes on and decide to do something more lucrative. Someone who takes a high-pressure job on high earnings may eventually lose interest in money in favour of quality of life. Wherever you are in life, think about the balance you have struck between wealth and happiness.

How would you describe your current financial/material situation?

- More than enough
- Enough
- Less than enough

How would you describe your current levels of happiness/contentment?

- Very happy
- Moderately happy
- Less than happy

Would you be willing to trade in some money for more happiness, or some happiness for more money?

Adapted from *The Money or Your Life* by John Clarke.

There were three reasons for putting money first in this book. First, to bring it right out in the open and allow you to be both realistic and honest with yourself about its importance. Because our society has such an ambivalent attitude towards money, few of us are ever really honest with ourselves about the role it plays in our lives. The second reason was to start unravelling money from other things we value in life and work, in preparation for succeeding chapters. And the final reason was to put it to one side. There are more ways than one to make a living, and with the understanding that the need to earn is implicit, the rest of the book is devoted to helping you find the way that will bring you most happiness and satisfaction.

5

Why else do we work? Meaning

This chapter looks at all that work brings us in addition to money. By the end you should have a better understanding of:

- the balance you like to strike between freedom and obligation
- the benefits of work
- which activities at work you most enjoy
- the most important things to you in a job.

I've long been fascinated by the phenomenon of the rush hour, and there's no more striking illustration than watching people walk over London Bridge. Between 8 and 9 every weekday morning thousands upon thousands of people, all dressed in suits, all carrying briefcases and umbrellas, walk northwards over the bridge from the railway station to the City. And between 5 and 6 every evening they all stream back again. For the most intelligent and self-defining of species, it's a very humbling sight. We've explored one of the reasons we are prepared to behave in this way, but if money were the only reason, we'd be in a sorry state. This chapter explores the others.

Slave or free agent?

A 'slave' is defined in the *Oxford Dictionary* as 'a person who is the legal property of another, servant completely divested of freedom and personal rights', while the word 'free' is defined as: 'Not in bondage to another; without ties, obligations, or constraints upon one's action'. There's a great deal of positivity in our culture attached to the word 'freedom' and a great deal negativity attached to the word 'slavery'. So much so that you could be forgiven for thinking that everybody's quest in life is to leave anything remotely resembling enslavement as far behind as possible and rush towards freedom with the greatest of speed. The strange thing is, most of us opt for a life that lies somewhere in between.

Think of all the areas where we voluntarily give up our freedom in return for other benefits. We give up the freedom of being single, for example, to be in long-term relationships. We do that for stability, to provide for children and to form relationships of greater depth and reward. While not everyone is willing to give up freedom of sexual partners indefinitely, there are few who wouldn't like their partner to do so. That's part of the deal. We also voluntarily give up the freedom to take other people's property, so they won't take ours; we give up freedom of movement to have a safe and regular place of residence; and we give up freedom of behaviour to be part of a cultural or religious group.

Ways in which we give up freedom

We give up freedom of:	In order to:	To achieve:
Time	Work	Money, etc.
Sexual partners	Marry	Loyalty
Location	Rent/buy housing	Stability
Actions	Obey the law	Order, safety
Children	Send to school	Education
Behaviour	Pursue religion	Eternal life

So although slavery as defined in the dictionary is thankfully rare now in Western society, there are a variety of ways in which we're far from free. One of these is obviously employment. When we're employed, we give up freedom of time and movement in return for money. If earning is a necessity and work a drudge, then a person may well feel enslaved. In these circumstances, freedom in the broader sense may simply be an interesting theory. On the other hand, if work is enjoyable and fulfilling as well as financially rewarding, then the balance starts to move away from slavery and towards freedom.

Freedom's just another word for nothing left to lose.
From the song 'Me and Bobby McGee' by Kris Kristofferson.

Thinking about the ties and obligations you have in your life at the moment, and of the freedoms you have, ponder for a moment where you feel yourself to be on that spectrum between slavery and freedom. Put your finger on the spot, or make a cross with a pencil. Now consider where you would like to be on that spectrum and, again, mark the spot.

Slavery_____Total freedom

Unless you're very unusual, both your crosses will lie somewhere between the two extremes, and the reason is that while freedom may be attractive, it has some rivals in our hierarchy of needs and desires.

Freedom has some rivals in our hierarchy of needs.

What does work bring us?

Structure

One of those rivals is structure. Many years ago I went with a group of friends to South Wales for a long weekend. One morning found us on the vast expanse of pale yellow sand that is Rhossilli beach, and there we invented a game. Based on many a team game, it involved a ball, two goals and two teams. We started in anarchic fashion, doing everything we could to put the ball into the opposing goal, but in no time at all we were making rules, setting boundaries and inventing sanctions. Why? Well, first of all, people started doing things we didn't like, such as tripping people up when they had the ball, and taking the ball and running off into the sea with it. Having outlawed these outrages, we then had to think of ways to continue the game after interruptions. Then we noticed we were all chasing after the ball but no one was there to defend the goal if the other team managed to break away with it. So we started to allocate roles to people. We were doing what has been shown again and again – put a group of people together for long enough, and they will organise and they will make rules.

The reason we organise is that we don't really like complete freedom all that much, especially if other people have it too. We prefer to have a framework within which we operate. We like to agree what we can and can't do in return for assurances that others will do the same. We like a little structure with our fun. You could go as far as saying that a little structure is vital to our fun.

Work gives us that structure. It gives structure to our days – how often do people express gratitude, if somewhat lukewarm, for something that 'gets me out of bed in the morning'? It structures our weeks. We know what we have to do on Monday mornings, and in return we are allowed to sleep in on Saturdays. It structures our years, which are punctuated by weekends, holidays and special occasions. Even our lives as a whole are structured by work – when we're young we go to school, when we're older we go to college or some other training, when we're older still, we go to work. And after a while, we retire. Work answers the question 'What shall I do now?'

The trouble is, every time we gain a little structure, we give up a little freedom. That's true whether it be work, marriage, games, religion, society or any other institution. The aim of good career development is to find a point on the scale between enslavement and freedom where you feel comfortable and happy, where the obligations and ties in your life are ones you take on willingly because they bring you something of value. The question is, what are those things of value?

For people who are in jobs they hate, who work for no more reason than having to earn, trying to think about what is good about work can be something of a trial. They'll be able to tell you with great fluency and conviction that work brings stress, tedium and terminal fatigue. That is work at its worst, and is as close as we get to slavery in the democratic world. But even in these unenviable circumstances work still provides money and still provides structure, and it may also provide a degree of identity and self-worth. At its best, work provides these benefits and a great deal more.

What does work bring us?

- Structure and routine (what shall I do now?)
- Identity (who am I?)
- Self-worth and personal fulfilment (am I OK?)
- Enjoyment (now can I have fun?)

Identity

For everybody, and I think it's safe to use that inclusive term here, work gives us an identity. It answers the question 'Who am I?' We tend to use the phrase 'I'm a manager, teacher, doctor, builder, solicitor, painter', rather than 'I manage, I teach, I heal the sick, I build houses, I advise people on the law, I paint'. In French, they drop the indefinite article altogether, giving for example 'Je suis medicin', not 'I am a doctor', but 'I am doctor', a much more self-defining way of expressing it.

Some will protest at the idea that they define themselves by their jobs, but like money and structure, you don't always realise the importance of something in your life until you no longer have it. Ask anyone who has been made redundant. Even if you don't define yourself by your work, it is difficult to get away from the fact that other people define you that way. Charles Handy, in his book *The Hungry Spirit*, tells of how he felt momentarily deflated when his young son reported having told the class that his father was a painter, having watched him decorating the house at the weekend. At the time he was a professor at a business school.

If you're in any doubt about the importance of identity in your work, try out a few different career titles for yourself. What would it be like meeting someone new and when they ask you what you do, you say, 'Well, hmm, I'm the prime minister actually'. Or 'I'm an artist', 'I'm a foreign diplomat', 'I'm a secretary', 'I'm a plumber', 'I'm an astronaut', 'I'm a housewife', 'I'm a neuroscientist', 'I'm retired, at college, unemployed', 'I don't have to work, I'm a millionaire'. See how you feel as you put on each of these identities and notice how the other person responds.

Self-esteem and contribution

Next, work of some kind is essential for our self-esteem and sense of contribution. It doesn't have to be paid work, but productive employment of some kind is necessary for us to feel good about ourselves, to be able to answer the question 'Am I OK?' in the affirmative.

It's relatively easy for healthcare professionals to see how they contribute, as they are there to help patients, but the kind of contribution varies substantially from one clinical area to another, as do people's ideas of what constitutes a contribution. I once saw a psychiatrist who had specialised in autism and finally given up because to her, the job was full of useless paperwork and devoid of the satisfaction of being able to help in any real way. We didn't discuss personality type, but this is a typical perspective of someone for whom the future is more important than the present (*see* Chapter 6). These kinds of people want a better future for their patients, and they deplore paperwork. Practical people who live for the present might see this job completely differently – as a way of helping families cope with autism on a day-to-day basis, of dealing with the practical issues competently and doing the paperwork that supported those activities.

Similarly, logical types like to contribute their competence, while 'people' types like to contribute their personal qualities. Organised people like to contribute their efficiency, while flexible types like to contribute adaptability and fun. Extroverts like to contribute their social skills and introverts like to contribute the fruits of their reflection.

So not only do we like to think we make a difference, but we like to think that we bring something special to a job, so that if we leave or go on holiday, they may cope without us but things will not be quite the same. Certain facets will be missing that only we bring. These are our qualities, and we like to use them and be appreciated for them.

I remember a time when my children were quite young when I went on a week-long residential course. This was the first time I had been away longer than a couple of nights since the children had been born. Now I love having children, but somehow a sense of identity as a mother was slow to come, and it was years before I stopped waking up in the morning surprised to find that I was one. Also, I selected a highly competent and willing partner who was perfectly capable of holding the fort, so I was not expecting my absence to be felt with any great force. Imagine my surprise, then, when I arrived home to somewhat unkempt-looking children who hurled themselves at me with unprecedented enthusiasm, and a partner who couldn't have looked more pleased to see me if I had been the allied forces arriving to liberate a prisoner-of-war camp. I have to confess to feeling ridiculously pleased.

Sometimes it's difficult to see how you make a difference. You have sobering moments, perhaps, when you wonder if anyone would notice if you weren't there, or when you think that anyone could do your job. If you do feel like this, it may not be because nobody would notice if you left, but because, like me, you have never stopped doing it for long enough. Or it may be that you're doing a job whose output you either don't value or don't realise, and you may not realise simply because nobody ever expresses any appreciation. There are some workers who are only really appreciated when they don't turn up. Think what the streets would look like if no one swept them. If you've ever experienced a strike of refuse collectors you'll know how appallingly smelly and inconvenient life is when they don't appear for a couple of weeks. On the other hand, there are people at the top of organisations whose absence, certainly for a week or two, would be barely missed. One might even go as far as to say that a good chief executive is one who only needs to pop in every now and then because it is everyone else who is carrying out the essential work of the organisation and they, like a navigation system, are only needed from time to time to check direction.

Think of the difference you make in your work. What do you bring that no one else does? What are you proud of? Who appreciates what you do? Who benefits? What would happen if nobody did your work for a couple of weeks? Who would miss you, and what exactly would they miss?

And where would our sense of self-worth be without human contact? Seeing other people is not just important for companionship, it's essential for our sense of who we are. We only know ourselves in relation to other people, can only assess our worth, our competence, our qualities and can only receive feedback if we are with other people. Even if you are in a job where regular conflict and ingratitude make you think you see far too much of the human race, it's likely that your patients or clients provide you with the highs of the job as well as the lows.

Making a difference, using our talents, being appreciated, human contact, all these feed our feelings of self-worth and personal fulfilment. Everyone values them, whether or not they are prepared to sacrifice them for other things.

Tied up with self-esteem and contribution is a sense of belonging. Some philosophers would say that a human being's main quest in life is to find a place where they belong, and in today's secular and divided society, work is probably the foremost provider of that sense.

Enjoyment

When, and only when, you have security in terms of who you are and how you matter, are you free to have that most cherished, yet most often sacrificed part of life: fun. To have fun you have to be spending at least some of your time doing things you enjoy. Even jobs with the narrowest of duties contain different kinds of activities and tasks, and for all of us there are some parts of our job that we prefer to others.

For many people the act of learning is fun. What is more exciting than being given the key to new information, new skills, new experiences of life? For some, activities that involve helping people directly are a major source of satisfaction, for others it is using their brains to solve problems. Some are never happier than when they are fixing things. Thinking about the activities you take pleasure in, and the specific aspects of those activities that give you satisfaction, can tell you much about what it is that you enjoy at work.

Many years ago I used to teach public health skills to medical students. People go into medicine for all kinds of reasons, but because we have so little experience of life when we're making early career decisions, much of our decision making relies on second- or third-hand information. In the case of medicine, a substantial proportion of this comes from the media, ranging from hospital soaps to news items. As you can imagine, medical students have much to learn about the reality of being a doctor.

Part of the students' course was to complete a project, and one group of students decided to look at patients attending the Accident and Emergency department and their referral to specialists within the hospital. This involved collecting data from a large number of patient case-notes. We met to discuss progress after they had been through the first 100. They were appalled.

It was so tedious! Did they really have to do any more? Was this really a good use of their time? This was their first lesson of working life. What they were thinking, but did not actually say, was that here they were, the cream of the British intelligentsia, doing the work of a clerk. Little did they realise that in among the healing and the caring, the heroic surgery and complex medication, the research and the innovation, is an entire continent of administrative work that has to be done. As our professor of pharmacology used to say to us medical students: 'All you need to be a house officer is a spinal cord and a pen'.

> *To judge a job on whether it contains tasks you do not enjoy is a recipe for long-term dissatisfaction.*

To judge a job on whether it contains tasks you do not enjoy is a recipe for long-term dissatisfaction. Can there be a job on earth that does not contain elements that one would rather not do? On the other hand, knowing what you do enjoy at work enables you to evaluate jobs both in terms of the proportion of time you are able to spend doing what you enjoy, and in terms of understanding how the less attractive aspects of the job support and feed into what you value about your work.

So what do *you* want from your work?

In this chapter, and the previous chapter, I've tried to gather all we value in work under a few general headings: money, structure, identity, self-worth and enjoyment. The headings are servants rather than masters, and the reality for each individual will obviously be more complex and less circumscribed. It is difficult to separate identity from self-esteem, for example, as each one feeds the other. Nevertheless, identity derived purely from a job would be a very superficial and vulnerable source of self-worth if it were not backed up with a sense of contribution and a feeling of affirmation from your fellow humans. Similarly money can lend a great deal to a person's self-esteem, but alone it's a very shallow companion. Enjoyment is enjoyment wherever you find it, but it's unlikely to lead to long-term happiness and satisfaction if it's not in tandem with a feeling that what you do matters. So the headings are not the whole story, nor are they mutually exclusive. They simply serve as a guide to areas you might like to explore when examining what is most important to you about work.

It's fairly easy to sit in the present and think of a few things you value in a job, but to find the real and full story you need to turn to your experience. If you've already done a number of jobs (paid or unpaid), think back and ask yourself 'What was the best job I ever did?' If you are early in your career development, ask yourself 'What project or piece of work have I most enjoyed? What did I most enjoy at school or college? When was I happiest, most fulfilled, having most fun?'

If there was a time in your life when you were really enjoying your work, think about what exactly it was about that time that made it so good. Was it the actual work? If so, what aspect of the work specifically? What activities did you most enjoy? (Use the list of work activities as a prompt.) Or was it your colleagues that you valued most? Or the working environment? Or the feeling you were doing something of value? Perhaps it was the autonomy? Or the support from seniors? Was it the challenge? The novelty? The variety? The learning? Looking at the headings identity, self-esteem, personal fulfilment and enjoyment, what did your best job supply in these departments?

What activities do you enjoy at work?

Practical tasks	Analysis
Technical tasks	Report preparation
People tasks	Managing budgets
Meetings	Bidding for money
Networking	Negotiating
Discussing	Organising
Variety of tasks	Speculating
Writing	Marketing/selling
Public speaking	Innovating
Teaching/training	Creating/designing
Mentoring	Having ideas
Problem solving	Motivating staff
Managing staff	Educational activities
Planning	Research
Strategic thinking	Brainstorming ideas
Implementing policies	Administration
Editing or checking	Counselling

Different facets of jobs can easily merge and blur in our subconscious, presenting themselves in our conscious minds as simply 'enjoyable' or 'not enjoyable'. Examining them in more detail can be very illuminating. For example, a scientific officer in pathology told me of a thoroughly rewarding job he had done a few years previously. In thinking about what specifically he had enjoyed, he started telling me about the technical work he had been doing. Then he stopped. 'Actually,' he said, 'I don't think it was the work that I enjoyed at all. It was the team. We all got on well together and it was great fun.'

Examining your worst-ever job in this way can be even more illuminating, as we often value things in life only when we no longer have them. It only takes an awkward colleague for you to realise the importance of congenial workmates. Or a boss breathing down your neck all the time for you to realise how much you enjoy autonomy and trust. Doing a repetitive and meaningless task may help you to understand the importance of intellectual stimulation, and a highly pressurised environment may bring you to realise how much you value peace and time for reflection. A job that ties you to an office or a desk may inform you that you would prefer to be out and about, meeting people or working in the open air. And one where the results of your work are all long term and difficult to define may tell you of a preference for immediate and tangible outcomes.

- What was the best job/work you ever did?
- What was good about it?
- What was the worst job you ever did?
- What was bad about it?
- What is your best kind of working day?
- What kind of people do you like working with?
- What sort of environment do you like working in?
- What specific activities at work do you like best?

When you have thought through the answers to these questions, draw up a list of the main themes that have emerged. What aspects of work are important to you?

1
2
3
4
5
6
7
8
9
10

For each item, ask yourself 'What do I mean by this, specifically, and what does it bring me in life?' For example, if you have put 'good colleagues', ask 'What do I mean by good colleagues?' Then ask 'What do good colleagues bring me in my working life? What are the benefits of good colleagues?'

Once you have a list, check for items that could be merged or modified. For example, you may have put 'learning' and 'intellectual stimulation'. Check if they are the same thing; if so, put them together. Aim for as concise a list as possible, and no more than six. List them below.

The most important things to me in a job are:

1

2

3

4

5

6

Now imagine doing a job in which you could have all but one of these things. Which one would you be most prepared to lose? Assuming you have six items on your list, put the number '6' next to the item you would be prepared to lose.

Repeat this process until you have prioritised all the items, and then write down your list in order of priority.

1

2

3

4

5

6

These are the things that are most important to you in a job.

How to feel free though tied

At the beginning of this chapter I explored the concept of slavery versus freedom. Although the *Oxford Dictionary* defines these words in absolute terms, in practice it is possible to feel free while you have ties and obligations, and it is possible to feel enslaved when you are technically free. How you feel about your life depends not on whether you are in work, but whether you want to be, and whether you want to be in that particular work. If work is providing you with good things you are unlikely to feel enslaved. You've given up some freedoms for a way of life you value and enjoy. If work is not providing you with those things, if it is unsatisfying, demoralising and unappreciated, then you may well feel enslaved. If it doesn't even provide you with enough to live on then you could argue that it is even worse than slavery. In these circumstances, you may crave freedom from your job, freedom to have a more fulfilling and enjoyable way of life, freedom to live.

The balance between enjoying work and wishing to be free of it depends not just on the nature of the job, but also on the other priorities in your life. Many people find that having children alters their attitude to work. Career women who never dreamt that motherhood would change their wish to work suddenly find themselves dreaming of working part time or giving up work altogether. Conversely, especially for men, children may mean an increased drive to earn in order to support them. Ill health, intimations of mortality and other life events can cause people to reassess their priorities, resulting in people dedicated to their work wanting suddenly to spend more time with their families, and those who have spent little or no time in paid work suddenly wanting to do so. The simple passing of time can also change our outlook on work, and something you found fascinating or exciting at 25 you may find unutterably dull at 50.

There is a quote bandied around which says that no one on their deathbed ever says 'I wish I'd spent more time at the office', but then again, I wonder if they ever asked someone who was long-term unemployed. Or someone who gave up their own dreams in order to support someone else's. Or someone who was unable to work because of disability or because they had a duty to look after dependants for much of their lives.

While many will fantasise about winning the lottery or making large sums of money in some other way, most of us do not have a comfortable private income, and for the majority who need some imperative to leave the warm comfort of bed in the morning, that is no bad thing. An irony of life is that while we all struggle to achieve freedom – freedom from poverty, freedom from want, freedom from bondage – without these apparently negative states there is little drive to do anything at all. A highly educated and intelligent friend of mine gave up work to look after her high-earning husband and three children. This was an entirely voluntary act and she enjoyed her life for many years. The trouble is, she told me, I never did anything work-wise because I didn't have to. Now, many years down the line, she wishes she had. Often the people who achieve most in life have been driven by some imperative – to escape poverty, please an unpleasable parent, fight discrimination, make a new start as a refugee in a foreign country. Adversity is a driver, as is want, and its value should not be underestimated.

If you do have to earn, the trick of a successful and happy working life is to have a job that gives welcome structure to your life, an identity you value, self-esteem and a sense of contribution, enjoyment and an income sufficient for your needs.

Oh, and one you can leave if you want to.

Work banishes those three great evils: boredom, vice and poverty.
Voltaire, 1694–1778

6

What sort of person are you?

This chapter looks at how the kind of person you are affects your working life. By the end you should have an understanding of:

- personality type and the meaning of 'preferences'
- your own preferences and personal style
- how knowledge of type helps in explaining past work experiences and in planning for the future
- what to do if you are in the 'wrong' job.

Mention personality types and people get nervous. Often there's a fear that if we start answering questionnaires on what we're like, all that careful work we've put into our outward appearances will be uncovered and we will be left naked in all our awfulness. And if it's not a fear of exposure that besets people, it's a fear of being boxed in. 'I'm an individual, how can I be put into a box with a whole load of other people?' they cry. Yet of all the techniques I use to help people understand where they are in their working lives, and where they need to go, increasing people's awareness of their personal style and preferences is one of the most powerful. Not only does it help in understanding why you enjoy what you enjoy at work, and why you do not enjoy what you do not enjoy, it also shines a light on relationships, working patterns, behaviour in groups, stress, strengths, what we find difficult, how we like to learn ... in fact just about everything in life.

The reason that a knowledge of your own and others' psychological type is useful rather than threatening, is that fundamentally we're all fine. We're only not fine if we conceal the best parts of ourselves, if we substitute our gifts with the qualities we think other people want, if we put ourselves not so much in a box, but in the wrong box. If you have ever watched people and wondered why certain things come naturally to some but not to others; why it is easy to communicate with some while with others you may as well be speaking a different language; or why certain types of people seem to congregate in, say, the caring professions while you find a rather different type in business and a still different type in academia, then this chapter is for you. If you have ever been in a job where you felt incompetent, undervalued, misunderstood, unaccountably weary or as if you are in a foreign land, then this chapter is for you too. Even if you have never been in these situations and are antipathetical to the notion of type, I ask you to come to this chapter with a sense of openness and a sense of curiosity as to whether the concept of type could be useful to you in developing your career and your life.

An introduction to Jungian typology

Carl Jung was a psychiatrist. In between all the theorising and philosophising and writing, he saw patients, and over many years of observing his patients he noticed that while everyone was unique, there were groups of characteristics that seemed to recur and cluster. He found that once he had some information about someone's behaviour and preferences in one part of their lives, he could predict their behaviour in other areas. He developed these ideas into a theory of psychological type that was published in 1921.

Around the same time, an American psychologist, Katherine Briggs, was pondering with fascination the differences she found between herself and her husband. There must be something really fundamental in people, she thought, to produce such different patterns of thinking and behaviour. When she read Jung's book she realised with great excitement that this was the answer she was looking for, and set out on a lifetime of developing his theory, joined later by her daughter, Isabel Myers. After decades of research, validation and refinement, the two women produced the Myers Briggs Type Indicator* (MBTI®), a self-administered questionnaire aimed at helping individuals find their type.

The theory of the MBTI® is that people differ in four main ways.

1   Where we prefer to focus our attention either in the outside world or in our heads.
2   The way we prefer to take in and process information; either literally and stepwise or generally and in patterns.
3   The kinds of information we tend to prioritise in decision making; either logical and objective or value-based and people-oriented.

---

*Myers Briggs Type Indicator and Myers Briggs are registered trademarks of the Myers Briggs Type Indicator Trust in the United States and other countries.

4   Our preferred style of living and working; either scheduled and organised or spontaneous and flexible.

These preferences all add up to a personal style, and it is this that the MBTI®
seeks to measure. Jung believed that preferences are inborn, but that the
extent to which we develop and express them is affected by our environment
and experience of life.

   Many will be sceptical of the idea that the human race can be encapsulated
in only 16 personalities, and of course they are right. Type is by no means the
whole story, it is simply a part of it that helps people to understand some of
the more fundamental characteristics. While the MBTI® has been validated
extensively through scientific research, the proof for the individual lies much
more in personal experience than it does in science. It is when you read the
description of your type and feel unnerved that a complete stranger could
know you so well that you are on your way to being hooked by type.

   The first step to experiencing the MBTI® is to understand what is meant
by 'preference', and the easiest way is to sign your name with your usual
hand, then do the same with the other hand. If you don't have a pen and
paper to hand, try clasping your hands together, interlocking your fingers.
Now clasp again, but this time have the other index finger closer to you.
Whichever method you use you'll find that the usual way feels easy and
natural, while the other feels awkward and difficult. The same applies to
behaviour preferences – you can do it either way, but one you can do
without thinking, while the other feels unnatural and you would probably
need to practise for a while before you could achieve anything approaching
the same result. It's not hard to imagine how difficult, time-consuming and
tiring it would be to have to use your non-preferred hand for writing all day.

Introversion and extroversion

The first of the four pairs of preferences is related to where you focus your
energy. When you are walking along deep in thought, not noticing the people
you pass, or the noise of the traffic, or the state of the weather, you are focusing
on your internal world (introversion). When you are talking with people,
attending to a practical task or physical activity, or noticing your environment,
you are focusing on your external world (extroversion). We all focus in both
places, many times a day, but we have a preference for one or the other, and
that place gives us energy, whereas the other takes our energy away.

   People who prefer to focus on their internal world, said to prefer introversion, tend to be the reserved, reflective people in life; the ones who like to
think things through before they speak or act, who prefer to spend time with

small numbers of people they know, and who find it easy to concentrate on solitary tasks. They tend to be energised by spending time alone or one to one, and drained by meeting new people and multiple activities. After a day of extroverting, which they may well enjoy if it doesn't happen too frequently, their idea of relaxation is likely to include solitude.

People who prefer to focus on their external world, said to prefer extroversion, tend to be the outgoing, action-oriented people in life; the ones who take initiative in social groups and at work, who are at ease with new people, who verbalise their thoughts as they are forming in their minds. They tend to be energised by active, people-filled days and drained by days sitting at a desk, studying or writing a report. After a day of introverting, their idea of relaxation is likely to include other people or activities.

Sensing and intuition

The next pair relates to preferences in the way we take in information. We all use both methods but some people prefer to take in information literally and chronologically, through their senses of sight, sound, touch and so on. These people, said to prefer sensing, are great on facts and detail, and they like to focus on what is, as opposed to what might be. These are the practical implementers in life, the ones who supply the detailed information required to make a pragmatic decision, who can be relied upon to give clear, step-by-step instructions for a given task, and who are able to experience and enjoy the present without worrying unduly about the future.

There are other people who also take in information through their senses, but who tend almost immediately to form patterns and meanings from that information, so much so that they may not be conscious of the detail that underlies those patterns. These people, said to prefer intuition, are interested in possibilities more than actualities, in the future more than the present, who rely on their hunches but are unable to explain where they come from. They tend to take in and express information in a haphazard way that can be quite bewildering to someone who prefers sensing.

Thinking and feeling

The third of the pairs relates to the basis on which people prefer to make decisions. Some people prefer to stand outside a situation to make a decision. They use logical analysis to work out the advantages and disadvantages of different options, they may be seen as hard-headed but fair, firm but reasonable, and they are said to prefer 'thinking'.

There are other people who prefer to make their decisions on the basis of their values and the effect that a decision will have on the people concerned. They may be less concerned with what is logically correct than with what is important to them and others. Said to prefer 'feeling', they are seen as sensitive, compassionate and tender hearted. If asked for a preference between the words 'justice' and 'mercy', a feeling type is more likely to prefer mercy and a thinking type justice. We all use both forms of decision making, but we have a preference for one.

If, for example, a manager has to make a decision about making a member of their team redundant, a thinking type may look logically at who is the poorest performer or the person who will be missed least in terms of reaching targets. A feeling type is more likely to consider people's personal circumstances and may let someone go who they know will walk straight into another job, rather than someone who might have more difficulty. It's important to understand that both these ways of making decisions are rational, and we are all capable of using both, they are just based on different priorities and different sets of information. Of the four pairs, this is the only one where there is a gender bias, with around 60% of men preferring thinking, and around 60% of women preferring feeling.

Judging and perceiving

The final pair of preferences relates to how you like to live your life in the external world. If you are someone who likes getting things done, who likes their life to be largely scheduled and organised, who is more comfortable when a decision is made than when it is yet to be made and who feels the need to finish work before they can play, then the chances are that you prefer judging. (NB: Judging does not mean judgemental.) If, on the other hand, you like keeping your options open, are flexible, feel constrained by timetables, can happily play when there is work to be done and feel energised by last-minute pressures, then you probably prefer perceiving.

What might your preferences be?

In the box overleaf you will find the four sets of preferences listed together with some of their key characteristics. The aim of the MBTI$^\circledR$ is for an individual to assess their preferences in each and end up with a four-letter type, for example E (extrovert), N (intuitive), T (thinking), J (judging). Taking the MBTI$^\circledR$ questionnaire and spending time with a qualified advisor is by far the best way to find your 'best fit' type, but it is possible to get an indication this way, and by answering the questions that follow.

Typical characteristics of people with different preferences

Extroversion (E)
- outgoing
- prefers talking to writing
- tends to speak before thinking
- wide circle of friends
- may find it hard to focus

Introversion (I)
- reserved
- prefers reading and reflection to action
- tends to reflect before speaking
- small circle of close friends
- work alone contentedly

Sensing (S)
- focuses on practicalities
- lives in present
- likes facts
- likes information in stepwise fashion

Intuition (I)
- focuses on possibilities
- lives in future
- likes ideas
- likes information as 'big picture'

Thinking (T)
- logical and analytical
- objective
- seen as tough minded
- interested in cause and effect

Feeling (F)
- value driven
- subjective
- compassionate
- interested in effect on people

Judging (J)
- scheduled and organised
- likes completion
- meets deadlines in good time
- hates last-minute pressures

Perceiving (P)
- flexible and spontaneous
- likes to keep options open
- feels constrained by schedules
- energised by last-minute pressures

When trying to decide on preferences, many people will say they tend to behave in one way in some environments and another way in other environments. This simply illustrates how we are all capable of acting in each of the preferences. However, there are some circumstances in which we feel able to be ourselves and some where we have learnt to behave in other ways. It is how we behave when we are most able to be our 'shoes off' selves that is the most reliable indication of our preferences.

Some people find it easy to decide on their type, while others find it much harder. This will depend on how true to type a person has felt able to behave over the years, the extent to which other people have valued their preferences and, of course, type itself. For some types, ESTJ for example, the world tends to be a place full of clarity and certainty, where they are regularly rewarded for their preferences. These people will often decide their type in a matter of minutes. For others, particularly perceiving types, deciding on type is more difficult. While the world, and the workplace in particular, tends to affirm people with judging preferences, those with a preference for perceiving often feel a pressure to be judging in their behaviour. Add to this their preference for leaving their options open for as long as possible, and it may be quite a while before they are happy to decide on a particular type. On the other hand, some may be so relieved to find that there is an explanation for how they differ from others, that they are only too happy to choose. There's no compulsion or hurry to decide on type. What is more important is that a person only opts for a preference or a type where they feel comfortable and which helps them to understand themselves better.

When differences cause trouble . . . and how type can help

As has been said repeatedly, we are all different, and while variety is what makes life so interesting and exciting, there are times when differences can cause problems. This is especially so when people don't understand type, and there is no preference that doesn't have the potential to bemuse and infuriate someone of a different type. You only have to look at the meanings and connotations that 'Extroversion' and 'Introversion' have acquired over the past 100 years to understand that.

To an extrovert, introverts may be totally unfathomable. Why on earth do they not speak? Why do I feel like a gabbling idiot when they're around? What are they thinking? In particular, what are they thinking about *me*? The word 'introverted' has gained all manner of negative connotations down the years, coming to be associated with personality disorders and other forms of mental illness. Psychiatrists, interested more in pathology than normality, have tended to measure levels of extroversion and introversion on a scale of 'sociability'. In other words, being sociable (i.e. extrovert) is good, while being unsociable (i.e. introvert) is bad.

To an introvert, extroverts can be maddeningly noisy. They come out with half-baked ideas, take up all the air-time and seem to have terrible difficulty sitting still. 'If they would only shut up for two seconds,' they think, 'I might have a chance to give them the solution/idea/insight I've worked out.' Introverts can find it difficult to understand that when an extrovert says something they are sometimes only thinking aloud, and use the same quality criteria as they would to assess something they themselves have taken hours, days or even months to think through. Similarly, extroverts may only ascribe the importance to the utterances of an introvert that they would to their own, unaware of how long the thoughts have been incubating.

If there is one pair of preferences that causes more difficulties in communication than any of the others, it is 'Sensing' and 'Intuition'. Sensing types may find intuitives hopelessly impractical, lacking evidence and always coming up with pie-in-the-sky ideas instead of concentrating on the issues at hand. Intuitives may find sensing types infuriatingly nit-picking, constantly interrupting their wonderful ideas with tedious practicalities. Whereas a sensing person likes to receive instructions in clear, stepwise fashion, intuitives may supply instructions in vague, haphazard ways that are totally incomprehensible to sensing types. Because intuitives like to find their own ways of doing things, they may feel oppressed by the detailed instructions showered on them by sensing types.

Thinking types may be exasperated by what they see as the wishy-washy, touchy-feely approach to problems that feelers seem to have. Why can't they be rational for once? Feelers, of course, can be appalled by what they see as the thinker's complete disregard for other people's perspectives and feelings. Because of the association of thinking with being male, and feeling with being female, these are the battlefields of many a relationship.

And of course the preferences 'Judging' and 'Perceiving' cause all manner of problems when brought together, whether it be in the home or the workplace. A supervisor with a preference for judging may find managing a perceiving employee very stressful, not knowing until the last minute if they are going to meet a deadline. The perceiver, on the other hand, may feel oppressed by the judger's need to have tasks completed ahead of schedule, because they need the last-minute pressure to become energised.

My preferences are for introversion, intuition, feeling and judging (INFJ), and I once worked for a man whose preferences were for extroversion, sensing, feeling and perceiving (ESFP). My strength is in using my dominant introverted intuition for coming up with new ways to look at things, new theories to explain things and new ways of doing things. I like reflecting and writing and working closely with a few colleagues, and because I am a judging type I like to be in control of my own work and to know the associated time-scales in advance. My boss, however, liked to be out and about, meeting people and collecting data, and just couldn't understand why I would want to sit in my office thinking. For my part, his proclivity for leaving decisions until the last possible moment meant I was unable to plan my work, and I often found myself having to complete large pieces of work at a few hours' notice – something that comes naturally to perceiving types, but is a nightmare for people who prefer judging.

Now the fact that I understood the contribution of type to my situation did little to solve the day-to-day problems, but it certainly helped me to cope on a personal level, because when you understand type, several things happen. The first is that you realise the other person is not deliberately trying to annoy you, they're just like that. Next you realise that you might be just as annoying to them. Finally you realise that their annoying habits may actually be quite useful (*see* Box).

Seeing differences through the lens of type

Types who prefer:	*May be seen as:*	*Could be seen as:*
Extroversion	Annoying, noisy, preventing me from speaking	Friendly, initiators, useful as networkers
Introversion	Deliberately silent, unnerving non-contributory	Thoughtful, interesting, good listeners
Sensing	Nit-picking, unimaginative	Practical, good at detail, grounded
Intuitive	Impractical, 'all over the place'	Good at ideas, the big picture
Thinking	Hard-hearted, insensitive	Logical, will make difficult decisions
Feeling	Soppy, illogical	Kind, good with people
Judging	Rigid, controlling	Getting things done, good planners
Perceiving	Unreliable, disorganised	Flexible, spontaneous

How can type help career choice?

The assumption when using the MBTI® in career development is that one of the most important motivations for choosing a career is the desire for work that will permit maximum use of your preferred functions and entail relatively little use of your less preferred functions. When your work plays to your strengths, you achieve much with little effort and much enjoyment. When your work plays to your weaknesses, you feel weary and inadequate.

Perhaps an intuitive person finds themselves in a clinical area that requires attention to detail and gives little opportunity for finding creative solutions. Or a feeling type works in a laboratory and never has the opportunity to help people directly. Perhaps an introvert is stressed because they're in a post where there is a never-ending procession of new patients and they never get the chance to think alone, or an extrovert has to sit at a desk for long periods. There are people who are idyllically happy in their jobs, in which case their type and their work are likely to be well suited, and sometimes people who appear quite unsuited to their jobs have found a niche that allows them to use their preferred functions.

Although individuals will naturally be suited to some specialties and jobs more than others, it is important to remember that type does not preclude anybody from a particular occupation. After all, if people were simply not able to function outside their preferences, no one would ever end up in the wrong job. As everyone is capable of writing with their non-preferred hand, given practice, everybody is capable of becoming skilled in their less preferred functions. For example, a preference for perceiving is wonderful if you are working in Accident and Emergency, where the need to respond flexibly to unscheduled events is paramount, as in any job where adaptability and openness to change are more important than completion and organisation. However, many jobs in the modern world value a preference for judging. Most bosses like to feel that everything is under control, want deadlines to be met in good time and are comforted by a semblance of order. Open and flexible types, therefore, often learn to be organised. They adapt to a deadline-oriented climate, they learn to be punctual, to finish one task before they start another, and to file things in such a way that other people can find them. They do it, but it's hard. It takes much effort, and although it becomes easier over time, it is never their strong suit.

Similarly, feeling types working in predominantly thinking cultures, for example in surgery, will often learn how to think objectively and analytically and keep their values to themselves. Introverts would not survive long in a clinical setting if they didn't learn to be extrovert, and intuitives have to learn the importance of detail. Thinking types have to learn how to understand patients' subjective experience, and sensing types have to learn how to make sense of complex information that arrives in haphazard form. Experience in counselling health professionals in their careers has shown that in nearly every case the problems and dilemmas being faced can be explained by comparing the individual's type with the content and circumstances of their job. Sometimes the sudden increase in awareness alone can be enough to solve problems.

Using work preferences to clarify type

In the following section, look at the two statements and consider where your preferences lie between the two. Make a mark on the line to represent this.

Example
I like working in a team (E)_____X_____I like working largely alone (I)

I like working in a team (E)   _____ I like working largely alone (I)

I like days full of action (E)   _____ I like days when I have a chance to reflect, write or study (I)

I like practical work, requiring precision and using hard data (S)   _____ I like using data to draw out meanings and develop theories and possibilities (N)

I like to see short-term results from my work (S)   _____ I am happy with delayed results if I can see a longer-term vision (N)

I'm best at making decisions using logical, objective analysis (T)   _____ I'm best at making decisions based on what is important to individuals (F)

I like to be complimented on my competence (T)   _____ I like to be complimented on my personal qualities (F)

I like creating organisation and structure (J)   _____ I like being flexible and spontaneous (P)

I like to know what I am doing, and when (J)   _____ I like 'anything can happen' days (P)

I prefer it when I have made a decision (J)   _____ I like to keep my options open (P)

Look at your responses, and the descriptions in the box, and place a cross on the lines below, at the point that best describes your own preferences.

Extroversion	_____	Introversion
Sensing	_____	Intuition
Thinking	_____	Feeling
Judging	_____	Perceiving

My self-assessed preferences are: _ _ _ _
(e.g. I S F P)

If you feel yourself to be exactly at the mid-point between two preferences, simply represent this as, for example, E/I or S/N.

How to check the suitability of a job

The beauty of understanding type is that it gives you a framework, not only for assessing your current situation, but one that can be applied to any situation, both real and potential. Imagine, for example, a young doctor is thinking of going into general practice and he is wondering whether it will be right for him. He is an ENFJ, an extroverted, feeling type, with a preference for intuition and judging. He enjoys working with people, has a warm, outgoing personality, and an ability to see patterns and meanings in information, together with an eye to the future. He realises that working within a group practice will probably suit him very well (E). His ability to understand trends and look to the future would be very helpful in the longer term for strategic planning of a practice, or if he ever decided to become a manager. He needs to check carefully, though, what exactly he would be doing in the typical working day. A new general practitioner is hardly going to go straight into management, and it is likely that their early years will be predominantly clinical; and much of the clinical workload will be hands-on, quick responses to straightforward problems (S). On the other hand, the long-term relationship with some patients, and the complex clinical and psychosocial problems they can present, will be more rewarding for an intuitive type (N), and most practices will come to know the GPs who are good at these kinds of problems and those who are better at the more hands-on, short-term challenges.

An ENFJ will enjoy interacting with patients, but the unpredictable nature of the work may be a challenge. Judging types like to be in control of their workload, like to know when they are starting work and when they are finishing, and a very busy practice where the work is never finished is likely to be very stressful for them. What our ENFJ needs to do is experience the work in more than one setting, assess the proportion of time he will be spending on his preferred activities and how willing he is to deal with the less attractive parts of the job. If he decides to go ahead he needs to choose a practice where he is more likely to be able to control his workload and where his strengths are needed.

Let's look at another example. A science graduate is considering training in histopathology. She is an ISTP, an introverted thinking type, with a preference for sensing and perceiving. She is an excellent technician. With her well-developed analytical thinking skills and her eye for detail she is well suited to diagnostic work, and the solitary nature of much of the work will play to her preference for introversion. Also her perceiving preference will serve her well when it comes to responding to urgent requests. Looking up the hierarchy, though, she realises that senior officers do much more than shift the technical work. They have staff to train and support, they plan systems of reporting, they respond to new management directives and laboratory standards. She realises that she will need to work on her people skills to be an effective team leader, her intuitive skills if she is to develop systems, and her judging skills if she is to survive the increasingly controlled nature of laboratory work. Like our potential GP, she will need to examine closely the proportion of her time she will be able to spend doing what she is best at, and think about how willing she is to develop her non-preferred behaviours for the more senior roles.

Any of the preferences can cause problems in a job if there is a predominant requirement for the opposite preferences. For example, an extroverted feeling and sensing type (ESFJ) who had been training for several years as a researcher, came to a halt in his career when he found it impossible to write up his thesis. While the conducting of the research had required attention to detail and gathering data (sensing), working within a team and making contacts (extroversion and feeling), and good organisational skills (judging), the analysis of the data required his least favourite function – thinking. Drawing meaning out of it required his second least favourite function – intuition. And perhaps hardest of all, writing it all up required long periods of sedentary concentration (introversion). He found it increasingly difficult to sit down at his desk, knowing how inadequate he would feel when he did so, and eventually he realised that what he really wanted was a job in which he could interact with people and help them in practical ways. Clearly an earlier understanding of type would have helped avoid years of feeling inadequate in what was, he finally decided, the wrong career.

Sometimes, though, understanding why you are having problems can enable you to stay in a career which you might otherwise consider leaving. I once saw a young surgeon who was having difficulties in relating to some of his colleagues. He was an ISFJ, while research has shown that nearly 90% of surgeons prefer thinking. He felt his strength was in dealing with the personal concerns of clients and their relatives, but that this contribution was rarely valued. Once he understood why it was he felt so strange and inadequate, he felt able to remain in the specialty with the knowledge that he had something unusual and valuable to offer.

Similarly, a health service manager with a preference for extroverted intuition with thinking (ENTP) was concerned about his lack of competence at implementing change. He said he was good at having ideas (extroverted intuition) and people seemed to find his input useful, but he was useless at working out the detail of how to put them into practice (sensing) and it didn't seem fair to delegate work, simply because he didn't like it. Once he realised that having ideas was something he did unusually well and that there were other people for whom practicalities were a strength, he felt better about not being able to do everything perfectly and about giving tasks to people who had different talents.

Using the insights you've gained so far into your own type and how it affects what you enjoy at work, take a job that you've either done in the past or are currently doing, and assess the content of that job in terms of the preferences required.

Job/career . . . . Past/current/proposed

This career/job involves:

Working as a team (E)	_____	Working largely alone (I)
Days full of action (E)	_____	Days when I can reflect, write or study (I)
Practical work, requiring precision and using hard data (S)	_____	Using data to draw out meanings and develop theories and possibilities (N)
Work that produces short-term benefits or results (S)	_____	Work, often complex, that results in long-term or broad benefits (N)
Making decisions using logical, objective analysis (T)	_____	Making decisions based on what's important to individuals (F)
Work where competence is of great importance (T)	_____	Work where personal qualities are of great importance (F)

| Creating organisation and structure (J) | _____ | Being flexible and spontaneous (P) |
| Largely scheduled days (J) | _____ | 'Anything can happen' days (P) |

My self-assessed preferences are: _ _ _ _
Predominant preferences required: _ _ _ _
(e.g. E N T J)

When you've done that, think about how the content of the job matches up to your preferences and what insights that gives you about what you do and do not enjoy or find easy at work. Once you have gained an understanding about one job you have experienced, try another. Then, with a greater understanding of how your preferences affect your work, you may like to take a possible future career or job and assess the extent to which your preferences will be matched.

What to do if you find yourself in the wrong job

Given the combination of external pressures and the over-reliance on exam success as a guide to career choice, it is all too easy to find yourself in a job that predominantly requires the use of your less preferred functions. If you are in such a job you may:

- feel inadequate
- find difficulty communicating with co-workers
- see problems and priorities differently
- feel you speak a different language
- find your strengths are underused and/or undervalued
- feel stressed, dissatisfied or weary.

So what can you do if this happens? Well, as with the young surgeon I spoke of earlier, once you understand why it is you are having problems at work, that alone may be enough to help you recover your confidence and your pleasure in the job. You may also be able to improve the situation through:

- working more productively with colleagues through understanding their preferences and using your own preferences in ways that complement theirs

- working on your non-preferred behaviour where the job requires it
- finding or creating a special niche for yourself where you can use your preferences productively
- volunteering for the tasks that are consistent with your type
- finding a home for your preferences outside work, for example in your leisure activities.

If all else fails . . .

If none of this works, you may be tempted to conclude that this area of healthcare is not for you, and you may be right. You may even think that healthcare as a whole is not for you. However, it may be that it is not the work but the people who are causing you a problem, and perhaps you just need to find an organisation or department where the culture is more in line with your preferences.

If you take dental practice, for example, there will be some practices where the predominant culture is sensing, and the attention is on using tried-and-tested techniques and doing them well. There will be other practices that have a more intuitive culture, where the treatment is more likely to be cutting edge and where there are possibilities to develop and change. Most careers require all the preferences, but while most workplaces would benefit from a good mix of types, in practice, people with the same preferences tend to cluster. You therefore need to look around for one where you will feel comfortable.

In summary, whatever problems you are having at work or in planning your career, and whatever solutions you have in mind, understanding how your preferences play into your feelings of satisfaction and enjoyment at work is invaluable for assessing current dilemmas and future options. Once you know what is causing you a problem in your current job or career, you will know what to look for in the next.

7

What's important to you in life?

This chapter asks you to consider what you value in life. By the end you should have a better understanding of:

- what is meant by 'values'
- what values your life currently reflects
- what really is important to you
- why knowing what is important to you is essential for planning your career.

There's a simple trick to life: know what you want, notice what you're getting and simply adjust what you do until you get what you want. What could be easier?

We all do this quite naturally when we're learning a skill. For example, say you were learning to play a forehand in tennis. You'd start with a clear idea of the result you wanted from your forehand: for the ball to go over the net and land in court. To begin with the ball will probably land in the net, beyond the back line of the court or even in a neighbouring field. But occasionally the ball will go over the net and into the court, and you'll start to notice that when you keep your eye on the ball, follow through with the racquet and keep your head down the chances improve. On the other hand, when you forget to watch the ball, worry about what the people on the next door court are thinking and swing wildly with your racquet, you'll notice that the chances of the ball going into orbit increase substantially. So you start consciously to do more of the things that work and less of the things that don't, and gradually your shot improves.

Similarly, managing work and life is a skill that can be learnt. But before you can do that you need to know what you want. Because while the game of tennis has very clear rules and boundaries, and simply watching it a few times will tell you that the idea is to get the ball over the net and into the court more often than your opponent, the rules and boundaries of work and life are much less clear. Even the criteria for winning and losing are surprisingly vague.

This chapter takes a look at what is important to you in life. You may wonder how this is relevant to the many practical and pressing issues that are facing you in terms of your work, but often it's the very assumption that work and the rest of life are two separate things that causes the problems in the first place. And even if that assumption isn't the cause of the problem, it has the capacity to make it a great deal worse.

What are 'values'?

If you are part of an organisation you may be familiar with the phenomenon of the 'away day', those days when the entire management board disappears to some secret venue in the country. You may wonder what on earth they *do* at those expensive country hotels for all that time. And frequently the only tangible product of several thousand pounds, a whole day and a combined IQ of several thousand is a sentence, intriguingly called a 'mission statement'. What, you may ask, is this ridiculous thing?

Well, strange and profligate though it may seem, there is some logic to this activity, because from time to time an organisation needs to check that its high chiefs have some shared idea of why they are all there. The mission statement of an organisation is an expression of its greater purpose, the reason it would like its employees collectively to rise in the morning, an expression of what it feels or thinks is important. It is an expression of its values. And the reason it takes a whole day away from the coalface to find and express these values is because, like castles built by children on the beach, the people have trampled, the wind has blown and the tide has come in so many times since they were first conceived that, often, there is barely a trace remaining.

It's the same whether it be an individual, an organisation, a country or the United Nations. The fundamental purpose of that unit's existence, something it seemed to know instinctively in its youth, tends to become subsumed over time. If you know what's important to you, and are living your life in harmony with those values, you can safely skip over this chapter, but if the last time you saw your values was in your teens it may be time for a little excavation.

If the last time you saw your values was in your teens it may be time for a little excavation.

The natural development of values

In *Zen and the Art of Making a Living*, Laurence Boldt talks about three different kinds of value: universal values, cultural values and individual values.

Universal values

Universal values are the ones that unite us all: love, peace, joy, health, nature and so on. That the plays of Sophocles or Shakespeare or the stories of the Brothers Grimm can speak with relevance to our lives today tells us that there are, at the core, certain timeless constants to the human condition. We don't tend to hear our politicians debating whether peace is a good thing, just whether another value, say freedom, is more important.

> The captain on a battleship spotted a small vessel in its path on the radar, and sent a radio message: 'Change your course!' The response came back 'Change *your* course!' The captain, exasperated, repeated the message. The same response came back. The next message to bounce over the waves was, 'I'm a battleship! Change your course!'
> Came the response, 'I'm a lighthouse.'
> Primary source: *The Daily Telegraph.*
> Secondary source: *The Magic of Metaphor* by Nick Owen.

Cultural values

Cultural values are the generally agreed upon social values of the day. They are the values held by the family, organisation, profession, class and country you are living in, and are concerned with ethics, manners and customs. Unlike universal values, cultural values change over time. For example, in the West, the past 50 years have seen major changes in attitudes to gender, the nuclear family and class. Cultural values pervade every aspect of our lives. They are so pervasive that most of the time we are not even aware of them, only noticing them when they are challenged in some way. Cultural values are at play when we wait in a queue, eat at table, choose what to wear in the morning, greet people, go shopping. They are the unwritten rules of society, and both insidious and invidious for that, for they mark you out as either member or interloper.

Values and medicine

In the early days, the values of medicine were laid down by Hippocrates, and many of the original principles remain: the sense of medicine being a privileged and exclusive club, with clear entrance requirements, codes of conduct and expulsion for those falling short of its principles. It is these very same values that are being challenged by society today, and this in turn is shaking up the profession perhaps more than it has ever been shaken up. For what is being questioned is not just the way doctors do things, but the very heart of what they stand for. Our society no longer values the deal it made with the medical profession – that doctors assure competence and probity in return for the public's respect and trust. It has some new values of openness, public accountability and user involvement. It wishes to renegotiate.

In the workplace, these rules are rife. I was once visited by a teacher friend of mine, who had just been to a job interview. She told me how well the interview had gone, what had been said, how she talked of the problems in her current post and how at one stage she had cried. Now at this point I struggled. How to reconcile these two pieces of information? 'The interview went well' and 'I cried'. And in my struggle I uncovered an important unwritten rule in medicine, and in other parts of the healthcare system, and that is: Thou Shalt Not Cry. Preferably never, and certainly not in interviews.

If you think there are no unwritten rules, try going to work in your bathrobe.
Laurence Boldt

Unwritten rules are the invisible walls that make it harder to succeed if you are a woman in a male-dominated specialty, a working-class man in a hospital where all the top people went to a smart school, or from a country or ethnic group which is outside the mainstream. For outsiders these rules are like trip wires; you fall over and can't see what it was that tripped you up.

Individual values

Individual values are our private meanings. They arise from temperament and experience, and are reflected in individual goals, relationships, personal possessions and preferences. Thus some people are ambitious in their careers while others are ambitious in their private lives; some spend their hard-earned cash on smart cars while others spend it on holidays; experience might cause one person to associate learning with ridicule, while another might associate it with fun.

Personality type will obviously play a part here. People who prefer extroversion are more likely to value the facets of life that occur in the outside world of people, events, surroundings and activities. People who prefer introversion may place more value on internal, private activities and a few close relationships. People who prefer intuition will value ideas, patterns and meanings, while sensing types are more likely to value pragmatism, detail and the here and now. Feeling types will have people high up on their list of values, together with compassion, harmony and sensitivity, whereas thinking types will be drawn to logic, justice and competence. Judging types are likely to have some values relating to order and completion, while perceiving types will enjoy spontaneity and fun.

We all have some combination of the three groups of values, whether or not we are aware of them, and our lives are a reflection of them. Every time we make a decision we are expressing one or more of our values. And every time we express a value, our lives are subtly moulded to that value. Whatever your situation now therefore, whatever your choice of career, partner, home, car – all these have been chosen by you, consciously or unconsciously, on the basis of what is important to you. Now you might say that you haven't made all these choices, that your parents chose your career, or your partner chose your home, or your friends chose your car, but even if this is apparently the case, in going along with their views you have expressed the value of pleasing these people, or of avoiding conflict, or of the ease of letting others take charge.

Values are not straightforward. They mingle with each other, conflict with each other and hide behind each other. There are aspects of our daily lives we think are important, that we say are important, but our actions say otherwise. How many times do we make New Year's resolutions only to go back to our old ways before the first month is up? If we could have everything we wanted, we would happily take it all, but if we have to choose, then some things fall down the list. We prioritise.

Because much of this prioritising is unconscious, sometimes we prioritise things that we wouldn't if we were fully aware of what we were doing. For example, in practice, we may prioritise lazing in front of the television when we get back from work, rather than attending an evening class or having a conversation with someone we love, but when we ask ourselves which of these things is more important, we may well say that, of course, having that conversation is much more important. If instead of taking initiative in our lives we simply respond to its demands, we soon run out of time and energy for other things. This more or less ensures that the novel is never written, the restaurant never opened, the holiday never booked or that you never get home in time to kiss the children goodnight, see your friends or take your partner away for the weekend. It also ensures, of course, that you never get round to doing the groundwork and planning for your life and career that you are doing right now. Being proactive over your values is energy-consuming and requires discipline. It's hard work, but the rewards are enormous.

When did you last see your values?

The nature of life in the twenty-first century is that we are always rushing somewhere, doing something, filling our time. If you work full time, the chances are that your job not only takes up most of your waking hours but also impinges on your leisure time. Even if you're not studying for exams and manage not to worry about patients as you lie in bed at night, by the time you get home after a full day's work what are you good for? How many of us have gone back to work after a summer break full of good intentions to see more of our friends, go to the theatre more, take up the piano, write a book? How many send off for the prospectus from the local college of adult educa-tion and book one, two or even three evening classes? And how long is it before we arrive home one day, the long summer evenings having retreated into two, then one, then no hours of light, come in from the chilly autumn wind, flop into our chair, put on the television and think no, I really can't face going out again for my class in astronomy/French/pottery/jazz guitar?

Sheer physical and mental limitations are just two of many things in life that cause us to adjust how we live it. When we're fresh and fit, our energy takes us to all sorts of action and dream realisation. When we're exhausted and spent, suddenly warmth, comfort and ease seem much more important.

Sheer physical and mental limitations are just two of many things in life that cause us to adjust how we live it.

To find out what is important in your life, it seems sensible to have a good look first of all at what you prioritise in your life right now. What do you spend most of your time on? What occupies most of your thoughts? How do you spend most of your money? Where do you focus your energy? These are the things that you've decided, either consciously or unconsciously, are the most important things in your life at present. It may be that you would rather not, on reflection, be spending your time, energy and money in this way, but doing so clearly fulfils a need in you, otherwise you wouldn't be doing it. So ask yourself, what do these things get for me? Why do I do them?

What do you prioritise in your life?

What are your three most important goals in life at the moment?
On what five activities have you spent most of your time in the past month?
On what five areas do you spend most of your income?
What has occupied most of your thoughts in the past week?
How are these things important to you? What do they get for you in life?

Memories and dreams

Once you're clear about what you prioritise now, it's time to see if there are other things that are important to you, things that have fallen between the stools of dreams and obligation. If it's a long time since you thought about such things you can find some clues by going on an archaeological dig of your past. You may find sitting at a desk with a pen and paper the best way to do this, or you may want to record the exercise on audiotape or ask a friend to read it out to you. Whichever way you choose, sit back, take some deep relaxing breaths, close your eyes and cast your mind back to times when:

- you were most creative
- you were having the most fun
- you felt most passionate or committed about something
- you were most decisive
- you were most absorbed by something
- you felt the greatest sense of achievement
- everyone said you couldn't do it, but you did it anyway
- you were happiest.

Allow yourself the pleasure of remembering in every detail what these times were like. What was good about them? Where were you? How were you feeling? Who else was there? What do they suggest to you about what is important in your life?

I once said to a pharmacist who was managing the pharmacy in a large hospital, 'I'd like you to think of the last time you felt excited about something'. Young, hard-working and ambitious, she had reached a state of deep anxiety about her ability to cope with the pressure and expectations of her career. She looked at me, first with incredulity, then embarrassment. 'I can't remember a time,' she said, 'no, I really can't.' So I asked her what activities she used to enjoy. Again, she had great difficulty. With a little more coaxing, though, a smile started to form on her lips. A few moments passed, the lines on her face melted and she seemed to be picturing some long-forgotten pleasure. 'Dancing,' she said at last, 'I used to dance.'

Our dreams are another source of clues, because our dreams are full of what we would really like, but have decided is impossible. I once saw a man who had made a great success of stockbroking in Hong Kong. Having lived the fast and dangerous life of a large casino, he eventually burnt out, as many do. All his money had gone on high living and he found himself penniless, with an anxious wife and three young children. He was unemployed when I saw him, living on benefits and had absolutely no idea what to do or any inclination to do anything. I spent nearly three hours trying to help him find something, anything, he could feel enthusiastic about. Just when we were both about to give up, something registered in his face quite suddenly. 'Actually', he said, 'what I've always wanted to do is grow things.' For a few moments he was animated, picturing whatever image he had of digging the ground, planting the seeds, watching as green shoots appeared from the earth. Then his face fell. 'But I can't do that, can I?', he said.

What are your dreams? What have you always secretly wanted to do, but never thought you could? What single thing would you do in your life if you knew you would succeed? There can be few people who have not wondered what they would do if they won the lottery. What would you do, and how would you spend the money? What would you spend it on if it all had to go within a few weeks?

Consider all the questions in the box and see what you find on your back burner, the things you would like to do, and intend to do ... one day? What have you consciously or unconsciously decided is not possible? And then (and you might need a stiff drink for this one) ask yourself: how do your current three most important goals in life, how you spend your time and how your spend your money match up with the answers to the other questions?

Memories and dreams

- What did you enjoy doing as a child?
- What do you, or did you use to, love doing as an adult?
- When was the last time you did each of these activities?
- If you won several million pounds in the lottery what would you do?

- If you had to spend your winnings within three months, how would you spend it?
- If you had just six months to live, what would you do in that last six months?
- What have you always secretly wanted to do, but never thought you could?
- What single thing would you do in your life if you knew you could not fail?
- How do your answers match up with what you currently prioritise in your life?

If your three main goals at present are very different from what you have written for other answers, or if you would change your life radically if you won the lottery or had only six months to live, ask yourself what makes you lead your life as it is now? And if the first thing you would do if you won the lottery is to give up your job, what is keeping you in what is clearly the wrong job?

Often the reason people give for staying in unrewarding jobs is financial security, something that would not be important if they had £5 million in their bank account or had only a few months to live. Whatever we do in our lives, we do for a reason. The purpose of asking the questions is not to devalue our motives, but simply to become more aware of them, so we can examine and make conscious decisions about them.

> *If you would change your life radically if you won the lottery or had only six months to live, ask yourself what makes you lead your life as it is now?*

If you have found a mismatch between what you value and how you live your life, take your main reason or reasons for living your life as you do now, and ask yourself the following supplementary questions.

- What does the reason (e.g. financial security) bring me in life? (The answer to this will often reveal underlying values.)
- What other ways might there be to meet these needs?
- If there is anything more important to me than meeting these needs, what would it be?

Similarly, if you find you would not change your life much, ask yourself what are the reasons for keeping your life as it is now, what is right about it?

Transgressions

Another way of finding out what is important to you is noticing patterns in what upsets, annoys or unsettles you. Casting your mind back over the past few years and searching for times when you have felt bad about something will often tell you more, and with greater precision, about what is important to you than any of the good times. I know, for example, that I have an allergic reaction to people treating other people badly, simply because they know they can get away with it. I'm not keen on people fighting each other either, or malicious damage, or cruelty, or a host of other negative behaviours that most people would agree were undesirable. But none of them hooks my emotions more than somebody being rude to another simply because they are stronger, or more senior, or richer, or feel themselves to be in some way superior to that person. If I ask myself what value of mine is being transgressed when people behave in this way, I realise that a strong value for me is that people deserve to be treated with respect, whoever they are.

> *If you see somebody absolutely incensed over something, you can be sure that a core value is being transgressed.*

For some people invasion of privacy is a pet hate, for others it is infringement of freedom. Some people just can't abide unkindness or meanness, others inefficiency or incompetence. If you see somebody absolutely incensed over something, you can be sure that a core value is being transgressed. If you see somebody in abject distress, you can be sure they are losing something of immense importance to them. If you see somebody in ecstasy, you can be sure they are experiencing something they greatly value. Our emotions tell it all.

So what are *your* values?

The process of excavating your values can be as alarming as it is illuminating. If you've never thought about these things, or at least not for many years, uncovering your values can be as disorienting as discovering you have a close relative you never knew existed. One client reported sitting in her living room quite unable to think of what was important to her and wondering in sudden panic, 'Do I actually exist?' But if you take the time and considerable effort to think about these things, and keep posing the additional questions, 'What is good about that?', 'What is important about that?', 'What does that do for me?', you'll find that certain themes start to emerge, that certain kinds of experience make you feel good about yourself, certain kinds of situations make you happy and certain kinds of transgression make you angry or upset. Effectively you are sorting your life experiences into those that are important in some way and those that are not. The themes that emerge could be called your principles, the things you would fight for, make an effort for, the things that your life would be desolate without.

The juggler

You are trying to learn the art of juggling. You have an array of brightly coloured balls and you endlessly toss them into the air, but every time you grasp one, another drops to the ground, and every time you bend down to retrieve one, several more fly out of orbit. Your ability to keep them all in the air falls as panic mounts.

Then a wise and kindly soul arrives and gently suggests that you stop juggling for a moment. 'Just put the balls down,' they say, 'and have a good long think about what you are trying to achieve with all this juggling. Perhaps you juggle as a form of meditation,' they suggest. 'Perhaps to entertain? Perhaps because you just like to learn new skills? Maybe you juggle because it gives you a deep satisfaction to watch the balls fly endlessly through the air? Now check each of the balls, and ask yourself what does keeping this ball in the air get for me? And this one, and this one? How does this particular ball help me in my overall aim? Now choose the balls that you really need, and try again.'

And so you do this, and you realise that in order to entertain with your juggling, the number of balls is perhaps less important than the colour of the balls or the arcs through which you throw them. You realise that in learning a new skill, it may be that you need to start with fewer balls and then add more as your ability improves. And as for meditation, well perhaps there are easier ways that don't involve balls at all.

When you have done everything you can to work out your values, ask yourself the following questions.

- What are the five most important things in my life? (Could be family, fun, love, honesty, humour, intellectual stimulation, physical activity, nature, kindness, fairness, recognition, music, travel, helping others, etc.)
- What principles would I most stand up for in life?
- If I were to choose a cause to which I dedicated my life, what would it be?

Why bother?

You may ask, why bother with values – after all, you may have muddled along through life without being particularly conscious of them. The answer to this is that values provide a firm foundation to build on. Without them we are liable to lose our way or be blown off course by the first stiff breeze. If you're familiar with project work or research, you'll know that the first thing you need to do is set down your aims and objectives for the work. Why are you doing the work and what is it you are trying to achieve? What different steps do you need to take to achieve that aim, to satisfy the underlying motive? If you try to do a project without these steps, either you speed your way through it and risk ending up with nothing of value, or you find trouble and indecision every step of the way. After all, how do you plan or implement or assess the quality of a piece of work if you don't know why you're doing it? But if you've taken the time to think through a project and you then get stuck half way through and wonder what to do next, which of many paths to take, how wonderful it will be to be able to go back to your single page of aims and objectives and remind yourself what you are trying to do. Life and work are the same. Knowing what is important to you will give you a sense of purpose and a sense of who you are. Armed with this you are in a much better position to set priorities, plan, make career decisions and, perhaps most importantly, manage adversity. When everything goes wrong and you're in danger of losing your bearings, this is a time when a solid rock of your baseline values comes into its own.

Knowing what is important to you will also, by default, help you to clarify what is not. Being more aware, more alert to the values by which you live your life, you start to question your actions, your motives and your feelings, and gradually the important things in your life float gently to the top, while the less important ones sink slowly to the bottom.

And when that happens, the result is ... happiness.

> *Yet hold on to your beliefs, and stay true to your values, for these are the values of your parents and your parents' parents; of your friends and of your society. They form the structure of your life, and to lose them would be to unravel the fabric of your experience. Still, examine them one by one. Review them piece by piece. Do not dismantle the house, but look at each brick, and replace those which appear broken, which no longer support the structure.*
> Neale Donald Walsch

8

What's important *about* you?

.

This chapter looks at what is interesting and important about you and your current and potential contribution to the world. By the end you should have a better understanding of:

- your special gifts and talents
- where and to whom they are important
- how they relate to your personality type
- how they act as clues to purpose.

Although we live in a society that is consumed with achievement, status and material success, it is considered poor taste to mention anything good about ourselves. Ask someone where they live, what car they drive, where they go on holiday, and they will probably be quite happy to tell you. Ask them about their children and you may have to put up your hand in protest to stop the flow, as there are few things people like talking about more than the talents and achievements of their children. Ask them about their own qualities though, and most will be rendered mute and mortified. Little wonder that so many of us resort to the external signs of success to advertise our worth.

A football player was known to be very modest about his sporting prowess. Once he had to give evidence in court and he was asked, so you're a football player are you? Yes, Sir, he replied. You any good?, came the next question. He was silent for a few moments, and looked very uncomfortable. 'Well, yes,' he eventually admitted, 'I'm very good, probably the best in the country.' Afterwards his amazed coach asked him why he'd said that. Well, he said, I was under oath wasn't I?
Source: *The Oldie* magazine, November 2003.

Not only are people reluctant to tell you what is good about themselves; if you probe a little you will often find that it is not just modesty that forbids them from telling you, but ignorance. So unused are people to talking or thinking about their strengths that frequently they don't even know what they are. Yet without a clear idea of what is special about your contribution to the world, how can you possibly plan your career? How can you feel sufficiently confident to take yourself out into the arena of life and work, and offer yourself as someone of worth?

> *Without a clear idea of what is special about your contribution to the world how can you possibly plan your career?*

This chapter asks you to put aside both modesty and outward accessories for a while and consider in some detail the qualities and talents you have been given. It moves the theme of importance from what is important *to* you into that powerful yet uncomfortable realm of what is important *about* you. Once aware of your qualities you're asked to explore where you use those qualities, what roles you play in your life and to whom those roles are important. Finally we look at purpose. Is there such a thing as life purpose and, if there is, what might yours be?

A unique contribution

We know that everyone is different. We can see that everyone looks different, that no one behaves in quite the same way as the next person and that we like people for different reasons. And yet at a subconscious level, perhaps because the thought that we are unique is just too frightening and lonely, we tend to assume that we're like everyone else. If, in a group, we feel different, we are more likely to think there is something *wrong* with us, rather than something special, and even the most unusual people seem to convince themselves they are like everyone else in all but a very few ways.

> *Our deepest fear is not that we are inadequate.*
> *Our deepest fear is that we are powerful beyond measure.*
> *It's our light, not our darkness that most frightens us.*
> Primary source: Marianne Williamson.
> Secondary source: Michael Neil Coaching Tips, www.geniuscatalyst.com

Once I was giving a seminar on psychological type to a clinical team. Two of the group, a male manager and a female nurse, identified with the psychological types that are most common for men and women (ESTJ and

ESFJ respectively), constituting around 20% of the population. At the other end of the spectrum there was a female doctor who identified with one of the least common types, representing about 1% of the population (INFJ). 'So,' I said to her, 'if you've always felt you are different to other people then this might explain it for you.' She looked at me surprised. 'But everyone feels different don't they?' she said. I turned to the man in the most popular group and asked him, 'Have you always felt you were different to other people?' He looked completely perplexed. 'No,' he said, 'not at all.' I asked the same question to the woman in the most popular group and she looked similarly surprised. 'I've never really thought about it,' she said.

The same is true of talents and abilities. If someone has a talent for something, they'll often discount it as unimportant, assuming that everyone has it. When talking to a nurse manager recently about her work, she described an awesome ability to run projects. 'I'm impressed,' I told her, 'you obviously have a gift for project management.' She was amazed. 'But that's how everyone does it, isn't it?'

It's true that we all have much more in common with each other than we have differences. We all have one head, one heart, and need to eat and breathe to survive. Nevertheless, every single one of us has qualities and special combinations of qualities that are unique to us. Even if we are not aware of it, the people close to us usually are. In any group of people, whether it be a team at work or play, a group of friends, a family, there are different skills needed, different parts to play. Take a clinical department, for example. There's the person you ask about tricky clinical problems, the one who is good with relatives, the one who likes practical procedures, the one who's good at handling psychosocial problems, the one who sits on committees and networks with other departments, the one who comes up with new ideas, the one who sits and thinks through every decision in careful and practical detail, the one who knows everything, the one who plans social events and looks after the staff, the one who leads, the one you can always rely on, the one who makes sure birthdays are remembered, the one who makes everyone laugh. We'd like to be good at all these things, but in practice we major on a few, and these talents and strengths are more than likely to be reflected in our psychological type. For every type there's a dominant function, and this is what we do best in life (*see* Box overleaf and Chapter 6, page 66).

Think of any group that you are a member of – it may be a team at work, your family, a community group, a sports team, a group of friends – and ask yourself what part you play in that group. What do the other people in the group value you for, and how would the group be different if you weren't there? What would they miss? Once you've done it for one group, try another and another. How do you adapt to the needs of different groups? What qualities recur?

What different types do best (dominant functions of MBT® types)

ISTJ and ISFJ: Introverted sensing. Fabulous at noticing and storing detailed information, and putting it to practical use. The data stored by ISTJs are likely to relate to objective issues, whereas in ISFJs the data will tend to relate to people.

INTJ and INFJ: Introverted intuition. Great at seeing meanings and patterns in complex information, generating new perspectives and ideas, theories, models and abstract concepts. Thinking types will tend to focus on the objective, while feeling types will tend to be people-oriented.

ISTP and INTP: Introverted thinking. Wonderfully analytical brains that cut straight to the heart of problems and solve them with ease. ISTPs are interested in practical applications, while INTPs are interested in theoretical and conceptual solutions.

ISFP and INFP: Introverted feeling. Deep sense of people-oriented values; work has to have a meaning. The sensing types live out their values in the present, while the intuitive types are interested in applications of their values to people's inner development.

ESTP and ESFP: Extroverted sensing. Energetic, in the moment, practical and realistic, they love to experience life and all it offers. They thrive in action-oriented work settings, where the work is varied and unpredictable.

ESFJ and ENFJ: Extroverted feeling. Warm and outgoing, they use their organisation skills to create happy, comfortable and harmonious situations for others (S) and a better world (N).

ENFP and ENTP: Extroverted intuition. Active, full of ideas for new projects, thinkers are systems and strategy oriented, while feelers are people-oriented.

ESTJ and ENTJ: Extroverted thinking. Highly organised, decisive and action-oriented, sensors are practical, while intuitives are strategic.

Some of our qualities we use regularly, and because they are such constant companions, we barely notice their presence. Others we may use less frequently, and if we leave them long enough we risk losing them. If you have excellent people skills, for example, but circumstances take you away from human contact for an extended period, or into a situation where others dominate, it might take a while for those skills to return when you are finally able to use them again. Similarly, an ability may become submerged if there is someone close to you who also has that ability and who is more dominant when it comes to using it. This is a phenomenon that has great potential in families and marriages. For example, if someone has a parent, sibling or partner who has a particular talent, they may hang back from using their own, for fear of negative comparisons. If using an ability seems to attract disapproval from others, rather than acclaim, that too may deter a person from using it.

If a quality or talent isn't used, it won't develop. Some qualities are innate and some are acquired, but even a Stradivarius violin needs to be picked up and played for its qualities to be realised. Drawing on your own experiences and your findings from previous exercises use the following questions to explore what talents and qualities you currently use, as well as those that may be hidden, unused, in your subconscious or your past.

What are your special talents?

- What part do you play in groups? If you're not there, what would be missing?
- Think of a time when you were at your best. Remember it in detail and ask what qualities were you exhibiting?
- What qualities do you most value in yourself?
- What qualities did you value in yourself as a child/teenager?
- What qualities do you most value in other people?
- What do other people (family, friends, colleagues) most value about you?
- Where do you currently use your best qualities?
- What opportunities does your current life present to use your talents?
- If there was one thing you would like to achieve with your talents, what would it be?

With all these questions it can be very illuminating to ask others what they think, especially if you have trouble coming up with answers yourself. And discovering the *differences* between what you value about yourself and what those close to you value can be especially interesting. Shelle Rose Charvet, in her book *Words That Change Minds*, talks about people who are internally or externally referenced. People who are internally referenced tend to have their own ideas about what is good or bad about themselves and will only accept outside views if they more or less concur with their own. For these people, the views of others are primarily matters of interest, rather than truth. Those who are externally referenced are more likely to look to others to discover what is valuable about themselves, and if those views differ from their own they are more likely to question their own judgement than that of the other person. To get a true picture, though, you need more than one view. If what you value about yourself is not what other people experience, then that is food for thought. Similarly, if somebody values you for a quality you were not aware of possessing, that too is food for thought.

Where do you use these qualities?

We bring our set of strengths and qualities to every role we play in life. If they seem useful and welcome in that role we use them, and if they aren't we try and develop the qualities we think we need. The average life comprises a surprisingly large number of roles. Most of us play the role of son or daughter for some part of our lives. Many will be brother or sister, father or mother, uncle or aunt, nephew or niece, husband or wife, cousin, grandchild, grandparent. At work most of us play the role of colleague, employee, friend or boss, sometimes all four at once.

Take a general practitioner (GP), for example. When he or she goes to work, they are a physician to their patients, a colleague to other staff, a teacher for juniors, a manager of a practice and a contractor with their local health organisation. But GPs don't just diagnose and treat patients. Patients need an ear for their problems, they need reassuring, supporting and comforting. Colleagues need mentors and friends, staff need support and appreciation. The practice needs running, developing and maintaining. Records need filing and organising. A GP has the opportunity to play any or all of these roles. Some they'll play more easily and more willingly than others, and their particular set of qualities will dictate what their patients and colleagues value and rely on them for.

Some roles may be less obvious than others, but if you carry out an activity you are playing a role of some kind. What role are you playing when you go for a run, for example, or cook a meal, or arrange an outing for colleagues? Who are you when you paint, sing, write, or play a game? Think about each role you play and how important it is to you. In what way are you important when you play that role, and to whom? What would happen if you stopped playing it, or if someone else played it? What do you do when you play the role, and which of your qualities are most useful or important?

What roles do you play in life?

- In what way is each role important to you?
- To whom is that role important, and in what way is it important to them?
- How do you play the role, and which of your qualities are most important when you do?

Most of us are unused to thinking about ourselves as important. Working through each role and its importance to other people helps to bypass those firmly entrenched aversions to self-glorification, operating as a back door to understanding the point of our lives as they are now. I once posed a question to a friend of mine, a kind and gentle woman totally devoted to her two children, who she looked after full time. What, I asked, would you feel about your children if you knew you were going to die? A sombre question certainly, but I wanted to discover what she felt about her role as a mother. So painful is the thought of not being there while your children grow up, most people would be unwilling even to contemplate the possibility, but my friend answered without a moment's hesitation, and with total certainty: 'I would wish they had never been born,' she said. This is someone with a perfectly good husband and no shortage of relatives and close friends, yet she was so sure of the essentiality of her role as mother, that she would wish her children had never been born rather than think of them growing up without her. That is importance.

As with talking about our qualities, our society doesn't really encourage people to go around thinking they are important. As children we loved to talk about ourselves and to be proud of our newly acquired skills, but how quickly we learnt not to do it with our friends. 'Boasting' is a mortal sin in the average playground, and claiming proficiency at a skill will ensure a large and avid audience, united in the hope that you'll fail. As a product of this culture, I'm sure that if I'd asked my friend what she thought was important about her, she would have blushed and not answered. But to feel that you matter is a source of motivation that we simply cannot do without, and it provides that most valuable of commodities, purpose.

In search of purpose

Examining the roles we play and the qualities we bring to those roles is a good first step on the road to purpose. Purpose is one of those private things that nobody speaks of. You can only surmise its presence when you see someone pursuing a goal with great determination and drive. Like the fellow diner watching the eponymous couple in the film 'When Harry Met Sally', when faced with these individuals one is tempted to ask the waiter, 'I'll have what she's having'. For purpose is a wonderful thing. It produces energy and focus like nothing else. If you think of the roles you play and find one or more that you play with commitment, concentration and passion, the chances are that it's a sense of purpose that drives you. There are few things as exciting as the single-minded determination to do something, and do it well.

You may believe in such a thing as life purpose or you may not, but whether you are religious or secular in your outlook, spiritual or pragmatic in your philosophy of life, thoughtful or active in your lifestyle, is there anyone who doesn't have moments in their lives when they wonder what it is all about, when they long for some explanation, some meaning, some purpose for life? Those moments are more likely to occur when things go wrong, as they reliably do from time to time – when we fall ill, lose loved ones, relationships break down, jobs are taken away from us, when we grow old. In between times maybe we say 'Ha! What a load of claptrap! We're here, we live, then we die. What more do we need to know?'

> *Is there anyone who does not have moments in their lives when they wonder what it is all about, when they long for some explanation, some meaning, some purpose for life.*

This section is not aimed at persuading anyone to a particular way of thinking or living or believing. It simply explores the idea of purpose, and asks the question not 'Is there such a thing as purpose?' but 'Would it be useful?' In particular, would it be useful for planning your career?

Quite recently I had a revelatory experience. I was watching one of a series of television programmes about the history of the British Empire. They had reached the 1950s and were describing the political climate and events in the Mediterranean. I had always felt a sense of connection to those times because I was born in 1956, the year of the Suez crisis, and I was watching with great interest. The narrator was talking about 1955 and the archive film, incongruous as it often is, was of the bows of a large liner ploughing through the waves. This was the year *before* I was born, I realised, and I drifted off for a few moments, vaguely wondering to myself if I had been thought of at that particular point, had I been conceived? As I ruminated peacefully to myself I was suddenly overcome with the thought that there was a time I had not existed, a time when I had not even been thought of. And that led quickly to the thought that again, there would be a time when I did not exist. And in between here I was. THIS IS MY TIME.

As that dramatic thought took hold, there grew in me a sense of excitement, as if I had a small but crucial part in a very long play, and had only just realised that it is now that I am on stage. Not before 1956, not in 100 years' time, but *now* that I have to play the part, *now* that the spotlights are on me, *now* that everyone is watching.

We all know at an intellectual level that this is true for everyone. Of course. Yet to experience it is palpably different. It's like being half asleep, not knowing quite what you are doing or what you are doing it for, then all at once someone or something gives you a shake and you realise you are not dreaming, not sleep-walking, this is the *real thing*. We're all on stage right now. Our time is short and we have choices with how to spend it. Will we skulk in the shadows, mumble our lines and just bide our time until we can slip unseen into the wings? Or will we exhalt in the wonder of it, the bright lights, the beautiful sets, the story, the rest of the cast, the possibilities, the preciousness of it all ... because we know it is not for ever?

It would be great, wouldn't it, if we all knew exactly what we were meant to be doing with this time, why we are here, what it is all about. Wouldn't it be easy to plan our working lives? Some people seem to know from an early age what they want to do and devote their lives to doing it. Listen to any interview with someone famous and the majority will say that they always wanted to sing, dance, act, write, be the prime minister, and that the signs were clear at the age of three. One feels sure that Mother Theresa was tending poverty-stricken dolls in infancy, that Shakespeare was writing sonnets before he could walk and that Bill Gates was registering patents in kindergarten. If you are someone who has slid from dilemma to dilemma with no deep conviction about what you want to do, it can be very dispiriting to hear these people. It's hard not to feel envious, and it's hard not to feel that your own piffling abilities and what you might do with them are as poorly set jelly compared with these pillars of certainty.

> *Talent does what it can, genius what it must.*
> George Bernard Shaw

With feelings like this, looking for a Life Purpose, capital 'L' capital 'P', can be a very daunting way to start exploring what we are meant to be doing on earth; like contemplating the summit of Mount Everest from the lowest of foothills. Suppose we start from the less alarming premise that our purpose in life is simply to use our special combination of gifts as fully and as often as we can.

Gifts: the clues to purpose

Earlier in the chapter you'll have looked at the qualities you bring to the roles you play in life. You will doubtless have found that you're good at quite a few things – in my experience health services are full of highly talented people who could turn their hands to any number of jobs. But surrounded by other talented people, you may doubt that you have anything special. Maybe you have the drive to do something, but don't think you're up to it. Perhaps instead of seeing a single shining path when planning your career, you're faced with half a dozen unmade roads. These are the stories of most people. Most of us have not been delivered with a genius that demands to be used in the way a screaming child demands to be picked up. Even the inspiring tales of vocation you hear on chat shows depend at least as much on struggle, dedication and plain hard work as they do on genius. Really.

It has often been said that we all have a special talent, and that is undoubtedly true. But that talent may not present itself in a single brightly coloured package. It may come as a special combination of gifts, an array of different colours. It may be that our own unique talent is lying not undisturbed deep in our psyche, but in understanding how the talents we are already aware of can be blended or arranged together into an exceptional combination. If there is a purpose in our lives, and who are we to say if there is or there is not, then maybe the clue to it lies in that exceptional combination and the opportunities to use it that your life presents. It's perhaps the ability to spot these combinations and put them to use that is even more important than the qualities themselves.

> *It may be that our own unique talent lies not undisturbed deep in our psyche, but in understanding how the talents we are already aware of can be blended or arranged together into an exceptional combination.*

Michael Brearley, a world-class cricketer, was known in the end not for his sporting prowess, but for being the best captain the English cricket team has ever had. An able sportsman though he was, his greatest strength lay in a deep understanding of and sensitivity to the human psyche. This gave him the ability to gauge the mood of the team, to know when to intervene and when to be silent, when someone was open to learning and when they were not, and the precise point when normal inter-team banter slipped into the danger zone. He understood how people ticked and he used that ability in the particular setting in which he found himself.

Imagine for a minute ... that a higher being was responsible for putting you on earth. This higher being has a plan for the world and you were designed uniquely and perfectly to play a particular part in that plan. The being has access to unlimited talents, and when you were put on earth they carefully selected the talents you would need to fulfil your special role. The being then placed you on earth at exactly the right time, in exactly the right body and in exactly the right circumstances for you to fulfil that role.

Take a good long think. Think of the talents you were given, the place and time you were born, the circumstances you were born into, and the opportunities and experiences your life offers. If there were a planned purpose for your life, what might it be?

Cast yourself in a role

Whatever your disposition on the meaning of life, I ask you to suspend disbelief for a little while and just pretend you do believe that there is a purpose for your life. Just for fun. You may like to do this exercise on your own or with a friend, or record it on tape.

Choose one thing you would really like to do, one important thing that would make you feel your life had been worthwhile. It may concern your current career directly or it may not. It may be something you are doing now and would like to carry through or something you have always dreamt of doing but never thought you could. It may be something great or it may be something simple. It may be something serious or it may be unadulterated fun. It may attract fame and fortune, or it may simply attract the affection or gratitude of a few others. It could be anything, as long as it is important to you.

Now take six pieces of paper and in large letters write one of these words or phrases on each piece of paper:

- environment
- behaviour
- abilities
- beliefs
- identity
- greater purpose.

Find yourself a bit of space and imagine a long straight line on the floor. Arrange the pieces of paper along the line at spaced intervals. Remind yourself of the important role you would like to play in your life and take a few moments to imagine yourself doing it. Cast yourself in the part. This is a game, so feel free to imagine wildly and with no modesty whatever.

Now stand on the word 'environment' and imagine you are playing this part. Ask yourself: Where am I when I play this part? What sort of environment am I in? What can I see around me? Who can I see around me? Take as long as you need to imagine yourself really there, see what you see, hear what you hear, and feel what you feel.

Next stand on the word 'behaviour', and ask yourself: What am I doing in this environment? How am I behaving? What tasks and activities am I engaged in? Take your time.

Now stand on 'abilities' and ask yourself: What abilities or skills do I have that allow me to do these things in this environment? What natural talents am I using? What skills do I have, and how did I get them? Whose help have I enlisted? What am I really good at?

Now move on to 'beliefs' and ask: What do I have to believe when I am in this environment, doing these things, and using these skills? What do I believe about myself? What do I believe is important? What are my thoughts about what I am doing?

And on 'identity', ask: Who am I? When I am here, and doing these things, and using these skills, and having these beliefs, who am I? You may be yourself, you may be a teacher, you may be an inventor, an entertainer, a sage, someone who knows their purpose. You may even be a god.

And finally, on 'greater purpose' ask: What is my greater purpose in doing this thing? Who am I doing it for? How will they benefit? What is my mission? How am I contributing to the greater good? Again, take your time to really feel what it is like to have this greater purpose, and when you have as much intensity as you can, start to move slowly back down your line, taking this sensation with you. Take your greater purpose to who you are and pause for a moment. Then take your greater purpose and identity to the beliefs you have, then the talents and skills you have, the things you are doing and finally the environment you are in.

When you've done this ask yourself, would it be useful to believe in purpose?

9

What are your assets?

This chapter takes a closer and more detailed look at what you have to offer in the workplace. By the end you should have a better understanding of:

- what you have gained from your life so far
- your qualifications, abilities, knowledge and experience
- how to sell your best assets on a curriculum vitae.

The preceding chapters of this book are designed to help you get to know yourself better, to dig up, dust off and examine those ideas, gifts and values that lurk in your subconscious. In doing so you will begin to understand how all these things combine to form the unique individual that is you. In this chapter we start to add the more accessible information, the assets you have accumulated over the years, the sort of personal information you might want to put in your curriculum vitae (CV). This may sound straightforward, and compared to excavating your values or working out your life purpose, it usually is. However, when people start to list their assets, perhaps for a job application, they tend to be limited in their mental search by what they think is important or what others will think important. The danger of this is ending up with a list that centres around your formal education and work, while omitting the vast wealth of skills, knowledge and experience that you've derived from the rest of your life. Also, people are not always aware of gaining skills. You may learn to do something as a by-product of learning something else, and may not be aware of having done so. In the same way as able-bodied people don't pride themselves on being able to walk, you may have skills but don't consider them as such because you take them for granted or assume everyone has them.

The processes laid out in the pages that follow help you to put your life experiences to date through a fine sieve. As each of the processes has the potential to feed into the others, it is worth reading the whole chapter before starting on the exercises.

Your life to date

Take a large piece of paper and place it lengthways in front of you. Depending on how old you are and how eventful your life has been, you may like to take two or more pieces of A4 and tape them together. Draw a long horizontal line to denote your life, and starting at the beginning of the line on the left, write the word 'birth'. Then moving from left to right, write down every major landmark or change in your life in chronological order, from your birth to the present. Include any geographical moves, life events and changes in terms of education or job. Once you have your full history on paper, start with your early years and take a moment to imagine yourself back in the body of the younger you. At each stage ask yourself the following questions.

- Where am I?
- What is going on in my family, my education/work, leisure and social life?
- What am I experiencing and learning?
- What am I achieving?
- What are the expectations/influences on me?
- What choices am I making and why?
- Is there anything unusual or remarkable about my life at this point?

Your location has an enormous bearing on your experiences of life, your learning and, perhaps most importantly, the situations in which you feel comfortable. My first five years, for example, were spent in Malaya. My early memories are of heat and palm trees, rubber and tea plantations; of brown-skinned people and rickshaws; of rambutans and assams, cobras and water snakes. I've been back to the Far East several times as an adult, something I may never have done had I been born in the UK, and I have an affinity with that part of the world, a familiarity with expatriate life and an ease generally with long-haul travelling. Some places confer a strong national identity, for example Wales and Scotland, and that sense of identity can stay with a person wherever they go. A religion may be part and parcel of being brought up in a particular place, for example Catholicism in Ireland, Hinduism in India, Buddhism in Thailand. Spending your early years in the countryside can leave you with a life-long yearning to be back there, as with being brought up by the sea, in a city or in a particular country. These experiences all provide knowledge of and access to parts of life that would seem foreign to other people, and will have a bearing not only on your options, but the likelihood of your taking them up.

Your family is a major source of experience and learning, and the role you play in your family is likely to influence the role you play in the rest of your life. A child may learn how to be a leader of their siblings, a peacemaker, an entertainer, a fixer, a follower, a carer. A child's personality and how it gels with the rest of the family will dictate whether they learn to be quiet or noisy, conforming or rebellious, open or defensive. Once at school we add other experiences and influences, discover our strengths, receive feedback from non-family members, take tests and either pass or fail. We make choices in our friends and our playtime activities, start to learn about the world in more abstract ways, and find an affinity with some subjects and a difficulty with others. Perhaps most influentially, we start to find out how we compare to our peers and we experience expectations from our parents in terms of that comparison.

As we move through school these perceptions become increasingly set, and by the time we are choosing our subjects at around the age of 14, we have a fairly clear idea of where we sit in the pecking order, what we are and are not good at, and what choices are therefore open to us. At this stage the world has already told us what it thinks is important. You know very clearly that parents and teachers will be pleased if you do well in your chosen subjects, that your university of choice will accept you if you succeed in your exams and that you can feel confident if you are at the top of the class. What the world does not tell us in such explicit terms is the value of all the other skills we learn in the course of our young lives: how to get along with people, how to get the best from them, how to organise yourself, how to make choices, how to present yourself, how to operate within a family, a peer group or an organisation. Some people have disability to cope with, divorced parents, illness in the family, personal tragedy. Some are coping in a second language and in an ethnic minority. Others are dealing with being too short, too tall, too plain, too spotty, too clumsy. While these different experiences can cause enormous misery, they also provide tremendous opportunities for personal growth. Emotional intelligence is now thought to be a much more accurate predictor of success than intelligence.

As well as academic and personal experiences, at all stages in life we are participating in other ways – in sports, the arts, leisure activities, domestic responsibilities, social interaction. We may take part in community groups, voluntary work, political activities. We read and watch television, go to the cinema and theatre, listen to music and look at paintings. All these provide experience, knowledge and skills, and sometimes qualifications. As you take a walk through your life, take note of all these experiences, notice how they affect the choices you have made along the way, and how they have led you to where you are now. Notice, too, any emotions attached to different periods of your life, and how those feelings have affected your view of yourself and your options. What have been the peaks and troughs of your life, and what do they tell you about yourself, your strengths and your weaknesses?

The QuAKE Review

Having reacquainted yourself with your personal history, you need to take a structured approach to what you have gained as a result. The QuAKE Review looks at your assets under four main headings:

- **Qu**alifications
- **A**bilities and skills
- **K**nowledge
- **E**xperience

Qualifications

Looking at your time line, remind yourself of every qualification or objective sign of success that you have picked up along the way. These may be in the form of:

- certificates
- school exam passes and grades
- music/drama/dance exams
- sports medals, certificates
- prizes and awards
- entry to schools/college
- diplomas
- degrees
- completion of courses.

Make a list.

Abilities and skills

You now need to remind yourself of all the abilities and skills you have found yourself to have naturally, or that you have gained along the way. Refer to Chapter 8 for your special gifts, and to your life history for skills you have learnt.

While there are some skills related to specific occupations, there are many that can be applied in more than one setting and some in almost any setting.

The demand and nomenclature for these skills, known as 'transferable skills', are subject to changes in fashion. In the 1980s, people were talking about supervising staff, in the 1990s it was managing staff and in the 2000s leadership is all the rage. In the 1980s, people were valued on their ability to meet deadlines, in the 1990s people would ask if someone 'delivered' and more recently people want to know if someone has good time management skills. Since Daniel Goleman had such huge success with his book *Emotional Intelligence*, there is a certain deference to the kinds of skills talked about in that book, in theory if not in practice, and 'good interpersonal skills' and 'excellent communication skills' appear in many a job specification. 'Team-working' is another term that is currently in vogue, as are 'motivation skills', 'appraisal', 'coaching' and 'mentoring skills'. Negotiation skills are much talked about in today's job markets, as are influencing and public relations skills. A familiarity and conversance with information technology is a must for a whole host of jobs.

Unless it applies to recent technology there is really no such thing as a new skill. All skills are old skills, they are just packaged differently, and the trick in self-marketing is to be aware of the current fashions and terms in the sector to which you are applying, and present your own skills in that way. Many of the terms are used simply to make the users sound innovative and interesting, but unfortunately they also have the effect of making people who are not up on the current language feel inadequate. If you are one of these people, remember the following.

- If you have ever thrown a party, you have leadership skills.
- If you have ever listened to a friend in need, you have mentoring skills.
- If you have ever shown someone how to do something, you have teaching and training skills.
- If you have ever given constructive feedback to anyone on a task they have performed, you have appraisal and coaching skills.
- If you have ever persuaded a child to do something they don't want to do, you have advanced negotiation skills.
- If you have ever written a letter that was understood, you have communication and writing skills.
- If you have ever worked on a task with someone else, you have team-working skills.
- If you have ever said anything at a meeting or a class, then you have public speaking skills.

Look at the following list and write a score between 1 and 5 against each one, where: 1 = poor; 2 = below average; 3 = average; 4 = good; 5 = very good.

	Score	Want to use	Want to develop
Establishing rapport with people	__	☐	☐
Networking	__	☐	☐
Keeping fit	__	☐	☐
Hand-eye coordination	__	☐	☐
Manual dexterity	__	☐	☐
Fixing things	__	☐	☐
Analysing data	__	☐	☐
Computer skills	__	☐	☐
Problem solving	__	☐	☐
Advising	__	☐	☐
Understanding people	__	☐	☐
Listening to people	__	☐	☐
Research and evaluation	__	☐	☐
Analysing options	__	☐	☐
Having new ideas	__	☐	☐
Inventing new ways of doing things	__	☐	☐
Seeing things in original ways	__	☐	☐
Developing theories	__	☐	☐
Making decisions	__	☐	☐
Using tools or machines	__	☐	☐
Caring for people, physically	__	☐	☐
Maths/statistics	__	☐	☐
Driving (car, boat, motorbike)	__	☐	☐
Sports	__	☐	☐
Assembling things	__	☐	☐
Analysing problems/situations	__	☐	☐
Finding out how things work	__	☐	☐
Reading or searching for facts	__	☐	☐
Committee work	__	☐	☐
Fundraising	__	☐	☐
Organising events	__	☐	☐
Self-awareness	__	☐	☐
Having insight/intuition	__	☐	☐
Implementing others' ideas	__	☐	☐
Playing an instrument	__	☐	☐
Editing	__	☐	☐
Composing music	__	☐	☐

	Score	Want to use	Want to develop
Selling/marketing	___	☐	☐
Explaining complex concepts	___	☐	☐
Painting, sculpture	___	☐	☐
Writing	___	☐	☐
Taking photographs	___	☐	☐
Making friends	___	☐	☐
Managing projects	___	☐	☐
Staying calm in a crisis	___	☐	☐
Playing a particular game	___	☐	☐
Creating a happy work environment	___	☐	☐
Interior decorating	___	☐	☐
Negotiation	___	☐	☐
Planning	___	☐	☐
Checking detail and accuracy	___	☐	☐
Managing money	___	☐	☐
Manipulating numbers	___	☐	☐
Drawing meaning out of facts/observations	___	☐	☐
Improvising/adapting	___	☐	☐
Leading	___	☐	☐
Making money	___	☐	☐
Team work	___	☐	☐
Setting up a business	___	☐	☐
Customer care	___	☐	☐
Getting jobs	___	☐	☐
Being interviewed	___	☐	☐
Interviewing	___	☐	☐
Assessing people's strengths	___	☐	☐
Teaching/training	___	☐	☐
Performing in front of people	___	☐	☐
Motivating people	___	☐	☐
Making people laugh	___	☐	☐
Mediation/diplomacy	___	☐	☐
Getting things done	___	☐	☐
Making new things happen	___	☐	☐
Communicating through speech	___	☐	☐
Self-motivation	___	☐	☐
Personal development	___	☐	☐
Writing action plans	___	☐	☐

	Score	Want to use	Want to develop
Inspiring love	__	☐	☐
Inspiring admiration	__	☐	☐
Perseverance	__	☐	☐
Planning strategically	__	☐	☐
Physical strength or stamina	__	☐	☐
Organising events	__	☐	☐
Administration	__	☐	☐
Dancing	__	☐	☐
Financial investment	__	☐	☐
Initiating	__	☐	☐
Completing tasks	__	☐	☐
Time management	__	☐	☐
Being positive	__	☐	☐
Being flexible	__	☐	☐
Planning systems	__	☐	☐
Entertaining	__	☐	☐
Multi-tasking	__	☐	☐
Being popular	__	☐	☐
Being precise	__	☐	☐
Seeing the best in people	__	☐	☐
Imagination and vision	__	☐	☐
Being flexible/adaptable	__	☐	☐
Inspiring people	__	☐	☐
Being wise	__	☐	☐
Being kind	__	☐	☐
Showing appreciation	__	☐	☐
Other skills	__	☐	☐

It's impossible to give a comprehensive list of all skills, so if you have some important skills that are not here, add them to the list.

Now take a highlighter and mark all the skills where you have scored 4 or 5. These are likely to be the areas where you have natural talent, and where acquiring skills therefore comes easily. You may already have identified talents related to these areas in Chapter 8, and they are likely to be connected with your Myers Briggs type. For each of these, put a tick in the next column if you would like to use the skill in the future, and in the final column, mark if you would like to develop the skill even more.

Now cast your eye over the remainder of the skills and highlight, in a different colour, any skills where you have scored 3. These are areas where you have adequate skills. While you may find some natural talents among these skills that your life has not so far allowed you to develop, these are more likely to be skills you have acquired, and are probably ones that you have found to be necessary in your day-to-day life. For example, you may not have a natural gift for using computers, but you may have reached an acceptable standard because you have found these skills to be essential in your work. Perhaps you are not naturally good with people, but have learnt to improve in this area because you realise it is important. Organisation may not be your strong suit, but over the years you have become reasonably proficient in this area. Mark any of these skills that you would like to use in the future, and any that you would like to develop further.

Finally, scan through the skills where you have scored below average and notice your reaction to these. This is an interesting group, as within them you are likely to find some important subgroups. One group is the set of skills you find most difficult, the ones that come least naturally to you and that you would like to avoid doing at all costs. Just reading them may bring you out in hives. Relating back to Chapter 6, on personality type, you will find among these skills your non-preferred ways of thinking and doing things. If you prefer sensing, for example, you will probably find skills in this group relating to ideas and theories, and doing things in new and original ways. If you prefer intuition, you will probably find skills relating to detail and practical imple-mentation. If you prefer thinking, you may find skills relating to people, and if you prefer feeling, you may find skills relating to logical analysis or how things work. If you prefer introversion, you may find networking here, while extroverts may find reading or writing.

The skills that you genuinely find difficult will probably constitute the majority of items in this group, but there is a second group that it is important to tease out and identify, and these are the ones that represent your beliefs about what you are capable of (see Chapter 10 for more on limiting beliefs). They are the things you don't do because they don't fit in with your image of yourself, or they conflict with your values. You may not do them because they frighten you, or because it has never occurred to you that you might be able to do them. You may play an instrument, but it may never have occurred to you to try and compose your own music. Perhaps you have services or products to offer, but the thought of marketing them brings you out in a cold sweat. Perhaps you have never really tried writing or painting or dancing, because in your youth somebody said you were useless at these things. Some people will find public speaking here (too scary), personal awareness (too touchy-feely), networking (why would anyone want to speak to me?), leading (what me?).

It's of huge importance to recognise the difference between the things you genuinely find difficult and the ones you simply haven't tried. The first group gives you fair warning of areas of jobs you will find difficult, and enables you to decide which you need to work on and which you need to minimise in your working life. In the second group you may not only find areas where you are potentially gifted, but here may lie the precise things that are keeping you from the career and life you want.

Summarising your abilities and skills

Take a pen and paper and write down your abilities and skills under the following headings.

- Areas where my abilities/skills are above average.
- Areas where my abilities/skills are adequate.
- Areas I find genuinely difficult.
- Abilities/skills I have avoided because of my beliefs about them.
- Abilities/skills I would like to use in the future.
- Abilities/skills I would like to develop further.

Skills may be grouped in various ways, as the examples in the box below show.

O: Organisation (management, getting things done, action)
P: People (communication, caring, getting on with, persuading, leading)
PS: Personal strengths (personal development, being cheerful, being positive, staying calm in a crisis, being flexible, self-motivation)
A: Analytical (numbers, data, research, problem solving)
PP: Practical/physical (precision, detail, fixing things, using tools, manual dexterity, physical strength)
I: Intuition/innovation/creativity (ideas, possibilities, big picture)

Looking at the skills in the summary, mark each one with the appropriate letter, and ask yourself, in which group of abilities/skills are my main strengths?
In which areas am I less skilled?

Knowledge and experience

If skills may be picked up unconsciously, then knowledge and experience are even more prone to being acquired without our realising. As we go about our day-to-day lives we rarely take note of situations we are exposed to and say, 'Wow! That was useful experience, I must put it in my CV.' Yet our lives are so rich and diverse from cradle to grave, that even the experiences of siblings in the same family can be remarkably different when you take a closer look. Siblings may live in the same house with the same parents, but they have different positions in the family, they may go to different schools, geographical moves will have happened at different ages and had different impacts. Different talents will have led them to different choices in academic and non-academic subjects, and they will spend their time with different sets of friends. One child of a parent who is a keen cook will spend hours in the kitchen helping and learning, while another will take no interest at all. One child may admire an entrepreneurial parent, watching and taking in all they see, while another may have no interest in business whatever.

In working life, different jobs will offer special experiences and opportunities to learn. My first job after qualifying was as a medical house officer in Jersey, one of the Channel Islands. Fresh and keen from a London medical school, I was fascinated by the array of neurological problems that presented to the hospital. I would perform extensive neurological examinations on these patients, resulting in complex lists of differential diagnoses. On the ward rounds, though, the consultant would take no interest whatever in my detailed case presentations of rare neurological signs. 'Alcohol!' he would say. 'Intravenous vitamins please!' And slowly I learnt that the most common cause of being unable to walk straight in Jersey was vitamin deficiency, due to a combination of excess alcohol intake and poor diet. Because Jersey is a popular holiday destination, the influx of summer visitors brought other interesting experiences. There was only one acute hospital on the island, so there was no question of the hospital closing, and when we ran out of beds during the summer months patients overflowed into the corridors. I learnt how to treat sunburn, how to transfer a patient by plane and how sad it is to go on holiday with your newly retired spouse only for overeating, overdrinking and unaccustomed sex to result in taking him home in a coffin. Admittedly, I have never mentioned any of these experiences in a job application. But if I had ever applied for another job on a tourist destination island, it would certainly have been a bonus if I could have told the employers that I grew up and worked on a holiday island and understood the different pressures on a hospital in such a place: the special problems presented by tourists; the low-paid seasonal workers; the high consumption of alcohol and tobacco; the difference between the indigenous islanders and the expatriates.

Building on the previous exercises, consider your life history and what knowledge and experience you have gained at each stage of your life. You may have gained knowledge from living in a certain place, or from having a family member or friend with certain knowledge or experience. You may have gained unusual experience and knowledge from having had a particular kind of schooling, for example a boarding school, a religious school or a school with a special ethos, as in Steiner and Montessori schools. What have you learnt from your parents' occupations and interests? What did you watch them doing, and where did you go and who did you meet as a result?

Your work may have taken you into a particular work environment or sector. General practitioners may work in old people's homes, prisons or police stations. Occupational health nurses and physicians often work in the commercial sector. Many healthcare professionals do work that involves management, legal issues, health service politics, research, education, social services, the voluntary sector. You may have worked abroad, at different levels of an organisation (local/national/international) or in different sectors (public, private, voluntary). You may have been exposed to specialised aspects of a particular job, have played a significant part in clinical management, had a special responsibility for teaching, or worked with someone with unusual skills or knowledge. Perhaps you did some interesting holiday jobs before or during your years at university, or maybe you have an interesting sideline now, in addition to your main job.

Think about your leisure pursuits and interests and how these have exposed you to various experiences. A remarkable sporting talent, for example, can take people into a very different world from the one they grew up in. What must it be like for a young person growing up in a poor area of an inner city to be suddenly thrown into the world of international athletics, for example? Or for someone growing up in an isolated rural community to find themselves playing chess for their county or country?

The social class you grew up in will also provide a particular set of experiences. People growing up in a working-class family will always feel an affinity for people of that class, and understand its customs and beliefs, whether or not they remain in it. Similarly, people from families in more privileged social groups will have an ease in that kind of company, and an understanding of its values, whether or not they espouse them. Class is something we tend to take for granted as it is so integral to our lives and early experiences, and yet it is a very powerful source of experience and knowledge. Ethnic background and familiarity with different racial and religious groups is a similarly powerful source.

What else has your life brought you? Has it led you to speak different languages, to campaign for political parties, to raise money for charities? What bad experiences have you had, and what have you learnt from them? Being mistreated, for example, may have been traumatic at the time, but you will doubtless have learnt much about interpersonal behaviour and coping strategies, and grown stronger as a result. Similarly failing at something can bring much in the way of learning, as can illness, death, divorce and other crises. All this knowledge and experience adds up to the person you are today. You may not wish to sell yourself in the workplace as a victim of circumstance, but you can certainly sell the products of these kinds of experiences.

So what are your assets?

Imagine you were writing a curriculum vitae in order to apply for a job or position where it is important to sell many facets of who you are, not just your work record. For example:

- to be a clinical director or manager
- to be the medical adviser on an expedition to deepest Peru
- to be an aid worker in a war-torn country
- to become a mentor for other healthcare professionals
- to represent your profession at a national steering group
- to be a candidate for a political party
- to adopt a child
- to be a foreign diplomat
- to be an astronaut
- to join the forces.

You may like to choose one of the above or think up your own job or situation. It may be a job or career that you have secretly often dreamt of doing but never thought you could; a position that you would like to attain by the end of your career, or one that lies outside your main career aspirations. Write a personal statement in support of your application under the headings that follow. Remember, nobody needs to see this, so you can write whatever you like, and in as glowing terms as you like.

Personal summary

Write two or three sentences that summarise who you are and what you have done. This introductory paragraph will establish an immediate impression, so you need to take great care that it is the one you would like to make.

Main strengths

Next, write down your main strengths. These are the things you are most proud of, and that are the most valuable assets you will be bringing to the role.

Additional skills, experience and knowledge

Here you should list all the skills, experience and knowledge you have that are of relevance to this role, giving evidence and examples for each.

Qualifications and courses

These should include:

- main school exams
- university degrees
- prizes and awards
- certificates
- postgraduate qualifications and degrees
- courses attended.

Interests and other experience

There is no need to include an exhaustive list here, but do mention activities and experiences that demonstrate your breadth and commitment as an individual, and anything that adds an extra dimension to your profile. This section also shows that you have a life outside work.

Plans for further development

This section allows you to demonstrate that you are someone who is always developing, and also that you are aware of any gaps there may be in your training or experience and are taking steps to address them.

Example

A specialist registrar in gastroenterology is applying to be the doctor on an expedition to Peru. He has five years' postgraduate experience, membership of the Royal College of Physicians and is the medical advisor for his local rowing team, for which he also rows.

He considers the kinds of qualities and experience the expedition leaders will be looking for, and decides on: appropriate medical experience, knowledge of tropical diseases, good teamworking skills, good in a crisis, track record of coping in adverse conditions, physically fit, travel experience.

Personal summary

I am an enthusiastic and hard-working person with excellent clinical skills and a proven ability to work in a team. I have five years' medical experience, including acute medicine, accident and emergency, and general practice, have travelled extensively and am a keen photographer.

My main strengths

- I am an able clinician
- I get on well with people, and am both popular and effective as a team member
- I am physically fit
- I am calm and efficient in a crisis
- I am an experienced traveller and have a good knowledge of tropical diseases

Additional skills, experience and knowledge

- I have been medical advisor to my rowing team for the past three years
- I have been on two previous expeditions: a walking trip in the Himalayas, and a trip across the Sahara
- I have experience of working in third world countries (Kenya and India)

Qualifications and courses

- School exams and grades
- Degree and class
- Postgraduate degrees
- Management courses (details)
- Personal development training (details)
- Time management course
- Diploma in tropical diseases

Interests and other experience

- I am a keen photographer, and have won several competitions
- I row for my county team

Plans for development

I am planning a period of working for VSO between completing my training and taking up a consultant post.

If you have worked through this and the preceding chapters, gathered everything that you have to offer and can present it with conviction in this format, you will be amazed to find what a fabulous, gifted and accomplished person you are.

10

What lies between you and your ideal career?

This chapter is about how you hold yourself back in life, and what you can do about it. By the end you should have a better understanding of:

- how what you do in life is affected by what you believe is possible
- the origin of limiting beliefs
- your own limiting beliefs and what they are costing you
- how to change those beliefs into new, more useful, beliefs.

In his famous book on transactional analysis, *I'm OK, You're OK*, Thomas Harris describes a disheartening process. Children, the theory goes, learn at a very early age that their parents are magnificent, while they are anything but. The small child is dependent, inept, clumsy, and has no words with which to express or understand meaning. By the age of five a child has learnt the inescapable truth, I am *not* OK, and much that happens from then on simply serves to confirm that perception. By the time we get to our late teens and early adulthood, most of us have a well-nurtured belief that who we are is just not good enough. To cope with this we develop a concept of who we'd like to be, and this becomes what we present to the outside world, what Jung called the persona.

In my picture there is a vast outer and an equally vast inner realm; between these two stands the individual, facing now one and then the other and, according to mood or disposition, taking one for absolute truth by denying or sacrificing the other.
From *Modern Man in Search of a Soul*, by CG Jung

Once we are clear about how inadequate we are, we make a lifetime commitment to proving we're not; to our parents, our teachers, our employers, our friends, our partners and, for some people, the world. It is because of this underlying feeling of inadequacy that we are such fertile ground for other people's values, and why over the years it is so very easy to forget that we ever had values of our own. Integral to this is the sensitivity we have to any suggestion that we are not who we would like to be. So for the person who has set out to prove their competence, a comment from another suggesting they are incompetent serves as a mortal blow. Similarly, the person who sets out to be kind to everyone is devastated when someone suggests they have been insensitive; so too the macho man, if it is suggested he is weak. The need to maintain these images can be so great that many people simply avoid any situation in which there is a chance of being found out.

> *The need to maintain these images can be so great that many people simply avoid any situation in which there is a chance of being found out.*

It is in this place of inadequacy and vulnerability that we build up a host of beliefs that limit us in our lives; and it's these that occupy the gap between what is important to us and where we focus our efforts. It's here we decide 'I am not the kind of person who …' and 'I have no talent at …' and 'I will never be able to …'. It's here that our hopes and dreams hit the rocks.

What lies between people and their dreams?
Beliefs – the rest is commentary.

This can make gloomy reading, especially if you are already well on your way to producing the next generation of 'Not OK' children, but Thomas Harris urges us not to lose heart. Everyone, he says, goes through this process to a greater or lesser degree, even his children. The imbalance of power inherent in the parent–child relationship makes it inevitable. The theory behind transactional analysis, as with most schools of psychoanalysis, is that once you understand why you feel inadequate in certain situations, why you feel the need to pretend you are what you are not and why you suppress your own convictions, you can start making changes.

The intrinsic nature, and therefore the danger, of limiting beliefs is that they are blind spots. For the most part we are unaware of them. If this is the first time you have heard of limiting beliefs, you may well think you have none. They are also self-perpetuating. As with any prejudice or assumption, our sensory systems select information that supports our beliefs. So if our impression is that white vans are always driven by maniacs, we'll tend to notice the ones which are and discount the ones which are not. These hidden and self-perpetuating beliefs have a profound effect on our actions, our feelings and, ultimately, our success and happiness.

The chicken eagle

There was once a farmer who found an eagle's nest while out rock climbing. In it were three eggs and, giving in to temptation, he put one of the three eggs into his rucksack and took it home. He placed the egg in the hen house, and one of the hens sat on it.

In time the egg hatched, and the baby eaglet emerged into a family of chickens. The eagle grew and learnt how to be a chicken: how to cluck, how to scratch the dirt for food, and how to flap and fly for a few yards before crashing to the ground. At no point did it occur to the eagle that it was anything but a chicken.

One day, late in its life, the chicken eagle looked up at the sky and there, soaring effortlessly high overhead, was an eagle. Our chicken eagle gazed in wonder at the power, at the grace, at the magnificence of this creature, and asked another chicken what it was.

'That's an eagle', said the other, 'the King of the Skies'.

'Oh', said the eagle-chicken, and went back to scratching the dirt.

Primary source: Fr Anthony de Mello SJ, quoted in *Awareness, Fount*.

Secondary source: *The Magic of Metaphor* by Nick Owen.

Where do limiting beliefs come from?

Parents

As a parent myself, I'm reluctant to dwell too long on what a rich source of limiting beliefs parents can be. But none of us are immune to the experiences in our lives that produce limiting beliefs, and the fact that we are mostly unaware of them makes it so very easy to pass them on without even realising.

We derive a strong sense of what is possible from our parents, and in particular what is possible for us. How parents love to spot themselves in their offspring! What a thrill it is to see yourself replicated, and what a comfort it can be to know that you are not the only person on the planet that can't do simultaneous equations, and not only that, you can blame it on your genes. We hear our parents explaining a poor result in a maths test with 'Of course, I could never do maths, he's just like me.' And we hear the same explanation given for everything from a lack of sporting prowess to difficulty making friends. When you hear these explanations as a child, you develop a view of yourself and the world that says most things are outside your control. 'There's no point in trying at English because my father was never any good at it, and I'm just like him.' 'No wonder I'm nervous meeting new people, my mother's really shy.' 'My parents tell me I'm a slow reader, so I guess that's just how it is.' We hear from our parents what kind of person we are and what we are able to do long before we have a chance to find out for ourselves.

Along with their limiting beliefs, parents pass on their fears. There are many areas in which parents communicate their fears, but there is one overarching message, and that is: The World is a Dangerous Place. As Susan Jeffers comments in her book *Feel the Fear and Do it Anyway*, how often do you hear mothers calling out to their children as they leave for school, 'Take lots of risks today, darling!' On the contrary, the prevailing message from parent to child is eternally 'Be careful'. 'Don't ride a bike – you may have an accident', 'Don't cross the road – you may be run over', 'Don't talk to strangers – they may take you away', 'Don't carry that – you'll drop it', 'Don't run – you'll fall'. Above all, don't do anything that might result in hurt or failure. And when you go against their advice, what happens? Our minds full of terrible possibilities, of course we fall, we drop the vase, we hurt ourselves. Can you even begin to imagine what your life would be like if you weren't carrying all that baggage around; what you would do if you were never fearful?

Parents also act as the first and foremost role models in our lives, and the presence or absence of role models is a rich source of beliefs about what we think is both appropriate and possible. If you're a woman, for example, you probably didn't grow up with fantasies of being a lorry driver, and if you're a man your dressing-up box is unlikely to have included a nurse's outfit. If you are a woman and were brought up by a working mother, you probably assume that you will continue to work too. If your mother stayed at home, then you are more likely to see yourself doing the same at some stage. If you are a man it is highly unlikely you have ever considered being a house-husband, as very few men are.

Did you ever consider being an actor, admiral of the navy, concert pianist, shoe designer, professional footballer, high court judge, entrepreneur, neurosurgeon, tightrope walker? If these occupations have never occurred to you, or occurred to you briefly before being set aside as ridiculous, then they probably don't figure in your family tree. It is hard to believe, for example, that the propensity for stardom among children of celebrities is all to do with genetics. It has much to do with contacts, certainly, and ready access to information and skills, but it is also to do with what you believe is possible.

People in films and television look so very distant to those of us who have no celebrities in our immediate lives. But for the likes of Stella McCartney, George Bush Jnr and Sophie Dahl, fame and success is something they grew up with. They have no such barriers. They may take a look at fame and reject it, they may take a look at their own skills and reject the specific area of fame that their parents have enjoyed, but they are unlikely to be limited by the belief, as many of us are, that stardom is out of reach. They have a choice.

School

If parents are the richest source of limiting beliefs, then school comes a very close second. I talked to a young woman recently who went to a highly academic school that not only excelled in exam results, but in every conceivable activity from art to singing, drama to sport, and where all performance was measured and evaluated competitively. It didn't really suit me, the woman told me, because I'm not very academic. I ventured that she would never have been accepted into the school if she had not been highly academic, but it was too late. The damage had been done a long time ago.

There is hardly a person I know who has not developed major limiting beliefs about themselves courtesy of school. A medical friend of mine was told that he should not apply for medical school because he would never get in. I know a man who engages in wonderfully creative activities with his children, yet thinks he is unable to draw because a teacher told him so when he was ten. My father was told not to sing when he reached secondary school because he was 'tone deaf'. And that is just the non-academic subjects. How many more people believe they are hopeless at maths? That they don't write well? How many people leave school thinking they are hopelessly dim? What a way to start a working life.

This is rarely the fault of individual teachers. Teachers operate, like all of us, in a society where beliefs and expectations abound. It is a society where everything we do has to be good, where we cringe to hear someone sing out of tune, where only the best pictures can ever be displayed, only the highest grades in exams are of note. It is not difficult to imagine what these attitudes can reap in terms of limiting beliefs in the children of today, and the adults of the future.

Examples of individual limiting beliefs

- I can't draw, sing, dance
- I'm not sporty

Continued

- I'm no good at exams
- I can't speak in public
- I'm a slow learner

Society

And then there is the wider society in which we live. All of us, parents and teachers included, are a product of societal culture and its beliefs.

Many cultural limiting beliefs are based on the premise that there isn't enough – not enough time, not enough money, not enough intelligence, talent, skill.

Examples of cultural limiting beliefs

- A mistake equals failure
- You have to be lucky to be successful
- You've made your bed, so you have to lie in it
- Changing your mind is a sign of weakness
- It's who you know, not who you are, that determines success

---

Ourselves

It would be nice to blame all our problems on other people, but the truth is that we are adept at developing limiting beliefs all on our own. The most common source of these is experiences we perceive as bad. Sometimes they involve physical hurt, as in falling off a bicycle, sometimes they involve emotional hurt, as in someone criticising our performance, but generally they all come down to one thing: failure. When we fail at something we make a decision about it. Either we decide that failing is an essential step to success and we just need to keep trying, or we decide that we are no good and give up. Sadly, we more often conclude the latter.

Our other contribution is in nurturing the beliefs that have been handed to us. These beliefs cannot survive on their own. They need attention, tending and feeding, and like the most assiduous of gardeners, that is what we give them. To rid yourself of limiting beliefs you not only need to starve them, you first need to find them, and that in itself can be quite an alarming process.

A Sufi tale

One night a man was walking along the street when he came across another, on his hands and knees, apparently looking for something under the street light. 'What are you looking for?' he asked. 'I'm looking for my keys,' the other replied. 'Where did you drop them?' inquired the passer-by. 'Over there,' came the answer, gesturing a few feet away. 'So, why don't you look there?' asked the passer-by, puzzled. 'Oh, it's too dark over there,' came the reply.
(Traditional)

How limiting beliefs affect career development

It is not difficult to understand how limiting beliefs affect our lives and our careers. Let's take the example of interviews, a process that just about everyone goes through at some stage in their careers, and one which may be repeated many times in the course of a working life. Most people who seek help to improve their technique in interviews have some deeply unhelpful beliefs. Frequently, their whole concept of an interview is a battleground in which both parties are trying to win. The candidate is trying to answer the questions, while the interviewers are doing their level best to trip them up. This perception is often embellished with other destructive thoughts – 'I'm hopeless at interviews', 'I'm not up to the job', 'There are other people going for the job who are much better than I am', 'There's an internal candidate', and so on. If you go into an interview with these thoughts, you may just as well pop your head round the door and say that you've decided to withdraw. Because just look at the consequences. As the interview approaches:

- you believe your control over the outcome is slight
- you develop discouraging pictures in your mind as to how the interview will go, visualising a sea of hostile faces and how you will be unable to answer the questions
- you are distracted from preparing the content of the interview and suspect there is little point in doing so anyway
- you become very anxious.

The net result is that by the time you reach the interview you are a nervous wreck, and you respond by being defensive or combative with the interviewers, or quiet and hesitant. Your mind goes blank when questioned and you either stutter over the answers or babble in the hope that saying something is better than saying nothing at all. You are therefore quite likely to fail, and this of course is like giving an extra big dose of fertiliser to the original belief.

Spotting limiting beliefs

Once you have a grasp of limiting beliefs you can have great fun identifying other people's, and as with many subconscious drivers and inhibitors, it can be easier to spot them in other people than it is in ourselves. It is interesting, for example, that while parents hand on their own limiting beliefs without even realising, they can spot an interloper at 500 yards. So when their child says 'I can't', instead of agreeing with them, they encourage them to try, and use expressions like 'There's no such word as "can't"'.

Phrases that are indicative of limiting beliefs begin something like this: 'I'm not the sort of person who ...', 'I've never been able to ...', 'I'm hopeless at ...', 'It's impossible ...'. They are expressed not only as facts, but as eternal facts. It has always been this way, and it always will be. There is no room for negotiation in the expression of these facts, it is just how it is. Start listening to people talk and you will hear these phrases sprinkled in everyday conversation.

To spot limiting beliefs in yourself and others, look out for sentences starting with words like:

- 'I am not the sort of person who ...'
- 'I always ...'
- 'Everyone says I'm ...'
- 'My parents always said I was ...'
- 'I've never been any good at ...'
- 'It's impossible ...'.

When you begin noticing them in others, see if you can spot them in your own language, particularly when you are explaining something you've done badly. When you forget things do you tell people you have a memory like a sieve? When you lose things do you tell yourself how disorganised you are? When you go into debt do you sigh, I'm so hopeless with money? If you fail to get a job do you tell yourself that you're just not up to that calibre of job? Try the following questions, adapted from *Your Best Year Yet*, by Jenny

Ditzler, to dig deeper into your limiting beliefs. You'll find it most helpful if you write down the answers.

- In what aspects of my education or career am I not achieving what I want? e.g. getting jobs, passing exams, progressing, relationships, interviews, direction.
- What reasons do I give myself for not achieving in these areas? e.g. I'm not clever enough, I'm no good at interviews, I'm not the sort of person who ..., I'm too old, I'm too indecisive, disorganised, shy, lazy. Or, the world is unfair, I don't know the right people, people are prejudiced against me.
- Where did I learn these beliefs? e.g. home, school, social group, work, the media, conclusions from experience.
- What have these self-limitations cost me? List them all, e.g. achieving my potential, some great jobs, a lot of money, happiness, health, self-respect, job satisfaction, contributing my gifts.
- In what ways have I benefited from these limitations? (and we all have), e.g. safety, an easy life, avoiding rejection, avoiding responsibility, time to have fun, not having to face up to things.

What to do when you've found your limiting beliefs

Have a look at your answers and ask yourself which area of your career or life has most suffered from your limiting beliefs about it? If you could really move forward in one area, which one would make the most difference to you? Write down your most limiting belief about that area of your life, and take a few moments to see how you experience having that belief. How does it feel? What do you see or hear when you have this belief?

Now ask: 'What other reasons could there be for me not achieving what I would like in this area?' Aim to find at least five. For example, if you believe your failure to progress in your chosen career is because you are not clever enough, consider other possible explanations.

- You need to work on your interview/exam technique.
- You have not applied for enough jobs.
- The career is extremely competitive, and you just need to persevere.
- You've been working in the wrong organisation or department.
- Your criteria for progress are unrealistic.

Which of your explanations do you find most convincing?

But what if my limiting beliefs are true?

This is a frequent question. What if I really am too old, too disorganised, too dim, too inexperienced, too clumsy, too shy? What if the world really is unfair, prejudiced against me, geared to people with contacts? These are fair questions, and to tackle them you need to understand a fundamental concept, and that is:

> *To assess a belief you must ask not whether it is true, but whether it is useful.*

Take this belief: 'It is dangerous to cross the road', and ask yourself, 'Is this a useful belief?'

Well, if you are crossing a road where cars travel fast and there are no pedestrian crossings, then this is a useful belief. It is even more useful if the visibility is poor, you have difficulty walking or if you are a child who cannot yet assess levels of danger. If, on the other hand, you live on the island of Sark, where the fastest form of transport is a bicycle, then the belief may be less useful.

In your career, it is useful to know that there are areas where you are excellent, areas where you are average and areas you find difficult. Why? Because it allows you to capitalise on your strengths, be kind to yourself about your weaknesses and know the areas you need to develop. What is not useful is to decide that because you are a thinking type, you will never be any good at dealing with people, or if you are a perceiving type, you will never be organised.

Non-useful beliefs	Useful beliefs
I'm no good with people	I need to develop my people skills
I'm not an 'ideas' person	Sometimes it helps for me to work with an ideas person
I'm lousy at detail	I can handle detail if I need to
I'm hopeless with money	I need to improve my money management skills
I'm too old	My experience of life will help me progress quickly

If a belief helps you to move towards the kind of life you would like, or away from a life you don't, then it is useful. If a belief holds you back from the kind of life you would like, or keeps you in one you don't, then it is not. At that point you need then to ask the question: 'What would it be more useful to believe?'

When a particular belief has been your constant and faithful companion for many years, you may find this question perplexing. The idea that you can choose what you believe may be totally new to you. Nevertheless, ask yourself: if you had a chance of leaving your old belief behind, and taking a completely new perspective, what new belief would really make a difference? What would you need to believe to feel really empowered in this area of your life? Choose positive beliefs that describe means and processes, rather than ones that simply contradict the original belief.

For example, new beliefs to counter 'I'm not the sort of person who ...' might be:

- I have the ability to follow whatever career I choose
- if I persevere I will succeed
- I can learn from setbacks and see them as essential steps to success.

If you have difficulty in finding useful beliefs, think of someone who is successful in this area and ask yourself, what must they believe to be so successful? You might even like to ask them. What would it be like if you had the same beliefs?

Write down at least three new beliefs, and when you have them, imagine what it would be like to have each one, taking time to experience it fully. Select the one that would make the most difference to your life, making any necessary adjustments until it feels right.

Beliefs into reality

Changing a long-held belief about something is easier than you might think. Take the important area of your life, and look at your limiting belief about it. Now look at your life and consider the consequences of holding on to your limiting belief.

- What is your life like now, as a result of this belief?
- What will your life be like next year?
- In five years' time?
- In ten years' time?
- In fifteen years' time?

Think of every possible negative consequence and make it as bad as it could possibly be. What will you be doing, how will you be feeling, what will people be saying to you, what will you be saying to yourself?

Then consider how you would prefer your life to be in this area. What would you like to achieve, and what could you achieve if only you could go for it with confidence and enthusiasm?

Imagine that you now believe your new empowering belief, and look again at your life. What is it like to have this new belief? Where will it take you in five years' time? In ten years? Fifteen years? What will you be doing, how will people see you, how will you be feeling? Paint the most wonderful picture you can.

Now decide which one you want.

Part Three

Let's get practical

11

Making sense of it all

This chapter pulls together what you have found, and helps you make sense of what it means for your career. By the end you should have:

- a written summary of your findings from previous chapters
- an understanding of the implications of these findings for your career
- a list of options for your future career or job.

If you have worked through the previous chapters in this book one or more things may be happening to you.

- You have a new understanding of yourself and what drives you.
- You have a clearer perspective of your life and career to date
- You know more about what you have to offer in the workplace.
- You are feeling more relaxed and positive.
- You are including more of the things you like in your life.
- You feel more in control of your life.
- You feel more confident.
- You are experiencing feelings of excitement about the future.

On the other hand, you may be feeling bewildered and confused by what you have found. You may be wondering what you have been doing with your life up till now. Maybe you feel alarmed, rather than excited, by the options that are opening up. It may even seem quite attractive to shut the book quietly and go back to what you were doing before. However you feel, positive or petrified, if you have got this far the chances are that you have what it takes to finish.

The first two parts of the book help you access the parts of you that are usually hidden, the parts you have forgotten, or perhaps have never been conscious of. This is undoubtedly the hardest part, as it is like using muscles you've been hitherto unaware of, requiring skills and activities that are entirely different to the ones that depend on your conscious, logical brain.

The third part of the book is devoted to pulling these new ideas and thoughts together, and putting them to useful purpose. You'll still need your ability to be creative and to tap your unconscious, but this part of your brain will be teaming up with the practical, logical side of your brain that knows how to make things happen.

This chapter is a stock-take. It helps you to assess where you are now by asking three simple questions:

- What have you found during your explorations?
- What does it all mean?
- What are your options for the future?

What have you found?

This first step is to remind yourself of what you have discovered during the course of each chapter and summarise them in a usable format. If you committed the exercises to paper, this is the time to read through them again. While you remind yourself, think through the answers to the following questions, and write them down.

- *What do I want in my life?* Drawing on the values you explored early on in the book, remind yourself of what you enjoy and what makes you happy. Remember what you thought you would do with your life if you could do anything or if you had just six months to live. Add anything else you identified as important when you looked at what you want from your work, and when you explored how your personal style and preferences affect what you excel at and enjoy in life. What qualities, possessions, people and activities do you want in your life?
- *What have I been given?* Remind yourself of what you found to be important and special about you; your qualities and talents; the opportunities your life has brought, and still brings you; the people and circumstances in your life; and the skills, knowledge and experiences you have gained as a result. What gifts and chances have you been given?
- *What would I like to contribute to the world?* Given what is important to you, and the gifts and chances that life has brought you, what would you like to give to the world? If you were to use all your gifts to the full, what would you be doing with them and who would benefit? What grand purpose would they fulfil and who would you be as you fulfilled that purpose? How would you like the world to be different as a result of your life?

- *What advice do I give myself?* Drawing from the things that have gone well in your life, and those that have gone less well, what advice would you give yourself for the future? Remind yourself of the tips you gained from Chapter 3, and add any arising from succeeding chapters.
- *What belief would be most useful to me?* Remember the thoughts and beliefs that stop you from moving forward? Ask yourself, what single new perspective or belief would be most helpful to you in making your contribution, in following the career you want to follow and in becoming the person you want to be?

Finally, if there were one thing that you have learnt about yourself and your career that is more important than all the rest, what would it be?

What does it mean?

The three major facets of your life – your values, your strengths and what you would like to contribute – are really all you need to plan not only your career, but your whole life. When they are all present and correct they provide a framework within which you can operate happily, and in congruence with who you are. They are like a navigation system, providing direction when you are planning, and guiding you back to safer waters when you lose your way. If you are happy, the chances are that your life is providing you with at least some of the attributes you value, that you are able to operate within it using your strengths and that you are contributing in some way, however small. If you are unhappy, the chances are that one or all of these things are missing, giving these explorations of yourself and your life the capacity to shine a revealing light on just what they might be.

The second step of the taking stock process is to understand what these findings mean in terms of your career. If you are just setting out on your career, then you should now be in an excellent position to develop some well-founded career options and move forwards. If you are further into your career, and picked up this book when you realised something was wrong in your working life, you may find that this process has simply served to confirm that you are in the right line of work. You just needed to understand why, and to tease out what are perhaps minor problems from the fundamental good in your situation. Maybe you need to make some small modifications as a result of your findings, or to find a more congenial job in the same field. If, on the other hand, you have found more serious mismatches between your ideal working life and how it is now, then you may be looking at significant changes in your working life. Looking at your summary, ask yourself, what are the implications for my career, and what is it telling me to do next?

When a major change is needed one of the hardest parts can be reconciling what you realise is right for you to do with all the years you haven't been doing it. This is more likely to be the case if you have thoroughly subjugated yourself and your desires to outside influence and pressure, or if you simply landed in something because that was the way the wind was blowing at the time. While some people do just fine being blown by the wind and manage to derive value and enjoyment wherever they find themselves, for some the discovery that their lives could have been different is a startling and uncomfortable revelation. Perhaps they realise they've been doing a job for many years and hating it, and now they understand why. They feel hopeless and betrayed, like someone who thought they had a good marriage only to find that their partner has been seeing someone else for the past ten years.

Faced with this, it is all too tempting to deny what you have discovered. You tell yourself, with some relief, that this is a load of touchy-feely non-sense. You find a wealth of reasons why you have done precisely the right thing and another lorry-load as to why you are going to continue to do it. The trouble is, once you know what you should be doing it will always be with you, and this is true whether you are at the start of your career or some way through. You have probably always known, and have kept pushing it to the back of your mind. As one client said to me: 'I have always had the idea that I should be a leader of some kind, that I should use my gifts in some grand way to help people. But it has always seemed far too frightening. I couldn't do that! A leader? Me? But in my heart I know that if I don't, I will wake up in the early hours of one morning when I am 70 or 80 or 90 years old, and it really is too late, and I will know that I have not done what I was meant to do. I will know, and I will weep.'

Taking yourself forward to a time when it is too late to plan your career is an excellent way of increasing your understanding of what you would like to achieve. Imagine you followed your values, used your gifts, fulfilled your purpose and lived by your positive beliefs and tips. What will they be saying about you when you retire? Imagine you are at your own retirement party and ask yourself:

- What would I like to have achieved during my working life?
- What would I like my boss or colleagues to say in their goodbye speeches?
- What would I like the beneficiaries of my work to say?
- What is the legacy of my working life? What am I leaving behind?

Compare the answer to these questions with what you think people would say about you now. Imagine you were leaving your current job or college, and all these people were having their say about you and your contribution.

How do their comments match up with what you'd like people to be saying when you retire? Are you on the right track? What is left for you to do? What else do you need to pay attention to?

If the gap between where you are now and where you would like to be is in the order of the Grand Canyon, don't despair. The important thing at this stage is to have some vision of what and who you would like to be. Once you have this vision, not only can you start to pay conscious attention to the steps you need to take, but your life will start to mould itself around your vision, as if of its own volition. There is no one who can tell you exactly how this happens, but there are many who would testify to its truth. The adage 'think big, but act small' is excellent advice for career planning.

What jobs or careers could I do?

Given what you now know about yourself, you may be developing a clearer idea of the kind of career or job that would be right for you. What does all the work you have done on yourself tell you to do? If you had a hunch as to the right work for you, what would it be, and what would you do if you had no doubts about your ability to succeed?

When we're starting out in life our options are largely set out for us by others. At this early stage there are vast numbers of careers that never even cross our consciousness. As we make our choices and progress down our respective career paths, we may become more aware of what there is on offer, but the choices we've already made mean our range of options appears narrower and narrower. Often people well into their working lives feel a deep sense of frustration when they discover all kinds of careers they would have loved to have done, but never knew existed. We all encounter people in our lives who are engaged in occupations that have never registered in our minds, and some will engender the same feelings you experience when you're faced with a particularly appetising morsel of food just after you've filled yourself on a meal you didn't enjoy.

Added to limitations placed on us through sheer lack of information, are those we impose on ourselves by what we believe is possible, what we believe we are capable of, and what we think are the limiting factors in terms of our qualifications, knowledge and experience. All this is compounded by the belief prevalent in our society that you should choose a career early and infreqently.

The result of all these factors is that when people are wondering what to do with their careers they are usually grappling with a tiny number of options which they believe to be acceptable and realistic. The task may be to choose between just two or three careers, specialist areas within a particular career, or just between specific jobs. Sometimes people have choices to make within their current job, and very often what stimulates people to seek help with their career is a simple dilemma: to stay in a particular job or not. It can be extraordinarily difficult to see beyond these narrow parameters, but the consequences of not doing so are far-reaching in terms of future fulfilment and happiness.

Brainstorming your options

The idea of this exercise is to throw out all the old limitations and spread the net as wide as possible. You may well come back to your existing ideas, but not before having some pleasure imagining all the other possibilities, and not before understanding those existing ideas in a larger context. A useful premise with which to start assessing the possibilities in your career is that there are always more options than you think, not just one perfect solution for you, but many.

> *A useful premise with which to start assessing the possibilities in your career is that there are always more options than you think, not just one perfect solution for you, but many.*

To explore your career options, turn to the diagram of concentric circles in Figure 11.1 and draw them out on a piece of paper. In the smallest circle, write the main options you are considering at the moment. As you write them down, take a few moments to imagine yourself doing these jobs – where might you be, who you are working with or for, what hours are you working, what is the work like, how are you enjoying it, and so on.

In the next circle, write down any other possibilities that you have considered, however briefly, and again imagine yourself doing those jobs. Notice any emotional reactions as you do so – they are useful pointers.

For the outer circle, write down anything you have ever dreamt of doing for a living, and some that you haven't. To help you in this task you could try the following.

- Imagine you have six other lives to live – what would you do in each?
- Recall what kinds of people you've looked at and thought, 'I wish I could do what they do'.
- Ask yourself which professionals/workers you most admire.
- Think about which of your hobbies you would like to convert into work.
- Look at the list of career options at the end of this section for more ideas.

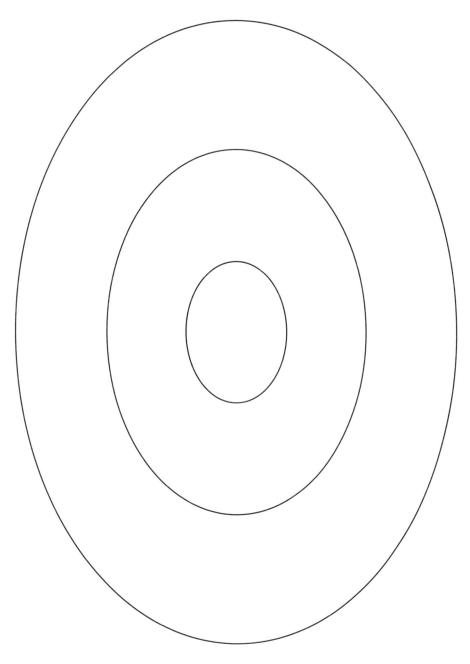

Figure 11.1

Write them all down and imagine doing them. When you have a good long list, look through all the options you've generated, and select the ones that you would like to investigate a little further. When doing this it is worth considering the following.

- If you have never looked into a career before you are unlikely to have a clear picture of how easy or difficult it would be to do, or how suited you are to doing it.
- You are not committing yourself to anything by exploring it.
- It is possible to have more than one career at a time.
- It is rarely too late to start something new.
- One of your options may be something you could take up as a leisure pursuit, rather than as paid employment at this stage.
- When you cross an option off the list, check your reasons for doing so. Life is not so cruel that we are given desires we have no hope of fulfilling. If there is something you really want to do, the only thing that stands between you and that career or job is your willingness to do what is necessary to get there.

Options for investigation

1
2
3
4
5
6

General career options

Management

- Public sector
- Private/commercial
- Industry
- Charitable organisations/voluntary sector

The law

- Solicitor
- Barrister

- Legal executive or clerk
- Coroner

Healthcare

- Medicine
- Professions allied to medicine (occupational therapy, speech therapy, physiotherapy)
- Nursing
- Clinical psychology
- Laboratory scientists and technicians
- Health service planning and development

Human resources

- Management
- Recruitment
- Training
- Career services

Art and design

- Painter
- Photographer
- Designer
- Stage production
- Theatre
- Film industry
- Copywriter
- Website designer
- Architect
- Publisher
- Musician
- Writer
- Actor
- Director
- Dancer

Retail

- Retail management
- Buying
- Training

Charity

- Management
- Fundraising
- Public relations
- Education

Media

- Journalism
- Public relations
- Broadcasting
- Script writer
- Researcher
- Editor
- Proof reader

Marketing

- Market research
- Training
- Sales representative
- Advertising

Self-employment

- Own business
- Freelance consultant

Education

- Lecturer/teacher
- Educational psychologist

- Health promotion
- Administrator/bursar

Politics

- Researcher
- Member of parliament
- Councillor

Academia

- Lecturer
- Research
- Laboratory technician
- Grant application and management
- Statistician
- Interviewer

Construction/technical

- Builder
- Plumber
- Electrician
- Surveyor

Computing

- Systems analyst
- Programmer
- IT consultant
- Website designer

Sports and leisure

- Professional sportsman or woman
- Training/coaching

- Providing leisure facilities
- Events management
- Travel agent
- Villa management
- Courier/representative
- Restaurant business

Other

- Finance and accounting
- Design and technology
- Secretarial
- Hairdressing
- Childcare
- Town planning
- Estate agency
- Estate management
- Urban regeneration
- Fashion designing or buying
- Manufacturing
- Civil service
- Library services
- Pet care
- Insurance
- Gardening/landscaping
- Farming/agriculture
- Counselling/psychotherapy
- Coaching and personal development

Options within medicine

Surgery

- Breast/surgical oncology
- Cardiothoracic
- Coloproctology and upper gastrointestinal surgery
- Ear, nose and throat (otorhinolarnygology)
- Head and neck
- Maxillofacial

- Plastics and reconstructive surgery
- Hands
- Neurosurgery
- Orthopaedics
- Trauma
- Transplantation
- Urology
- Vascular

Reproductive health

- Obstetrics and gynaecology
- Family planning

Anaesthetics

- General
- Intensive care
- Pain management

General practice

- General
- Academic

Internal medicine

- Audiological medicine
- Cardiology
- Care of the elderly
- Clinical oncology
- Clinical pharmacology
- Dermatology
- Endocrinology and diabetes
- Gastroenterology
- Genitourinary medicine (sexual health)
- Infectious diseases and tropical diseases
- Medical oncology
- Nuclear medicine

- Neurology
- Occupational medicine
- Ophthalmology
- Palliative medicine
- Renal medicine
- Respiratory medicine
- Public health medicine
- Musculoskeletal medicine
- Rheumatology
- Sports medicine
- Spinal cord injury

Accident and Emergency

Paediatrics

Diagnostic and interventional radiology

Psychiatry

- Adult
- Child and adolescent
- Old age
- Learning disability
- Psychotherapy
- Forensic
- Drugs and addiction

The armed forces

- Army
- Navy
- Air Force

Pathology

- Chemical
- Forensic
- Haematology

- Transfusion medicine
- Histopathology and cytopathology
- Immunology
- Medical microbiology
- Virology

Biological sciences

- Anatomy
- Clinical genetics
- Physiology

Complementary medicine (e.g. homeopathy, hypnotherapy, etc.)

Other career options where a healthcare background is either essential or useful

- Medical/health service management
- Medical/healthcare education
- Healthcare research
- Charities
- Medical ethics
- Defence unions
- Postgraduate medicine
- Teaching
- Medical IT
- Medical/healthcare associations
- Pharmaceutical services (advisory, publications, national bodies, government)
- Pharmaceutical companies
- Government departments
- Medical/healthcare journalism
- Prisons, police services
- Nursing homes
- Health-related broadcasting
- Management consulting in health services
- Non-executive positions

Self-employment

- Private clinical practice
- Consultancy
- Locum services
- Career development
- Writing
- Teaching/training

The importance of keeping your options open

There are stages in life when you have to make choices about your career, there is no getting away from it. This may be choosing subjects to study at school or university, choosing a field in which to train, choosing sub-areas of a particular field or choosing specific jobs. You are forced to choose because you are at a crossroads and standing still is not an option. Nevertheless, there are ways of choosing that reduce your options much more effectively and rapidly than others, and these are influenced not so much by what you choose, as by what you drop as a result.

Take the man who trains as a clinical psychologist, practises for a few years and meanwhile pursues an interest in athletics. At some point along the way he is given the opportunity to compete in athletics at a national level. This requires much training, and he eventually realises that it is impossible both to run his busy job and pursue athletics at the level he would like. Although he finally makes the decision to devote less time to work and more to athletics, he is still faced with a number of choices. At one end of the spectrum he could give up work completely and devote himself to his sporting career for the foreseeable future. At the other end of the spectrum he could simply modify his working life in order to shift the balance of effort more towards athletics. This may include reducing his hours in the current job, or changing jobs to one where there is more flexibility and less pressure to work long hours. In between these extremes, he could join a retainer scheme and give up, but only for a year or two, or continue working but in a different or limited capacity. The choice he makes will be dictated by a number of issues, including his values, his financial situation, how much he enjoys his work, the culture of his workplace and profession, and the needs and views of any partner or family. His choice will have a huge impact on his future career. The more he moves away from his work, the less likely it is that he will ever return to it. The more he keeps in touch, on the other hand, the more choices he will have when his athletic career slows down and he wants to return to more mainstream paid employment.

The same is true of a woman or man who decides to shift the balance of their life away from work towards caring for children. In this case, it is a question of 'when' and not 'if' they wish to return to some kind of occupation outside home, as children predictably grow up. While thoughts of returning to work typically occur when the youngest child goes to school, and again when the youngest leaves home, at any point along the way the impetus may be stimulated by divorce, financial problems or simply a desire to do something different. Many people who have been outside the workplace for a long time will respond to this urge by taking on activities other than paid work, but paid or unpaid, there are many more choices for someone who has kept up some extra-family activities.

While it is especially important to think carefully before burning your boats if you are considering giving up work altogether, the need to keep options open also applies to people who take up a career and pursue it for many years without break. There are few, if any, people who don't feel the need for change from time to time. Some may suppress this urge for a variety of reasons, but most will feel it. Among doctors, the number who choose an area of medicine early on in their careers and continue to do exactly the same work until they are 65 are very few indeed. A proportion leave medicine altogether early on in their careers. Some reduce their hours. Some change specialty. Some run into trouble and have to stop practising. Some leave through illness. Others take up medical politics, management, research, teaching and training, examining, writing or medico-legal work. Similar variations in career progression are to be found in nursing and professions allied to medicine, perhaps even more so. Human beings are programmed to desire change from time to time, and they may also be subject to change that is outside their control The fewer irreversible steps you take along your career pathway, the more options you will have when that change becomes either desirable or necessary.

And don't forget retirement. Sometimes high-earning people have the opportunity to retire early, leaving them suddenly with acres of spare time but with little practice in using it. If you go through life working every hour that is available, the thought of retirement can be terrifying. It is no coincidence that people who work till they are 65 have a much lower life expectancy than those who retire early. The move from continued employment to endless leisure is probably no easier than moving from being long-term unemployed to working again.

The key to healthy career development, therefore, is to balance focus with variety. You need to focus on a career in order to succeed, but you also need to keep options open for that time in the future when a particular job is no longer enough, or when it no longer wants you. So whenever you are taking an important decision about your career it is worth considering the following.

- Keep current channels open and maintain your skills in case you want to return to them later. If you are in a profession, check what arrangements are available for keeping in touch.
- Check your current career thoroughly to see if what you are seeking may be found within it. Most careers in healthcare offer many different facets.
- Combine your existing work experience with another. For example, our athletic psychologist might specialise in psychology as it relates to sport.
- Make change incrementally, rather than by quantum leaps.
- Pay attention to your leisure interests – they may lead to work, and they are invaluable for your happiness and sanity during the times you are not in work, whether through unemployment or retirement.

12

Getting motivated

Having options is nothing without motivation. This chapter looks at motivation. By the end you should have:

- a vision of where you would like to be in your career, and when
- an understanding of what you need to get there
- some resources to help you.

There was a time, many years ago now, when I was very keen to live and work abroad. I used to talk about this to my partner, who would nod in agreement, and I used to scour the back pages of the *British Medical Journal,* where the jobs in exotic locations were advertised. For a long time there was nothing of interest to be found, then one Saturday I opened the jobs section to find the perfect job for my partner in the University Hospital of Singapore. I was excited. I told him all about it. I sent off for the details (I know, I know). I made inquiries as to what work there might be for me. And all the while he nodded. The details came and he did nothing. I asked and I waited, and I asked and I waited. Nothing happened. Two, three weeks went by. One day I asked him, are you going to do anything about this job? He prevaricated for a while, but eventually he confessed that no, he wasn't. And the reason? He didn't want to work abroad. He may not have realised he didn't want to work abroad, but when it came to acting, the bit of him that knew better dug its heels in.

What do you need to move forward?

- To know what you want
- To understand what is needed to reach it
- To be absolutely sure that your desire to pursue a career is sufficient to outweigh the costs of doing so

Whatever you decide to do with your career, whichever of your options you choose, you need to be absolutely sure that your desire to pursue it is sufficient to outweigh the costs of doing so. No amount of knowing what to do will result in action unless you are motivated.

Take a walk into your future

This process is designed to inspire motivation by giving you a glimpse into the future. Taking you forward to a time when you have the career you want, it:

- allows you to experience just how good it is going to be
- shows you the practical steps that you will need to take to reach it
- enables you to give yourself some resources to overcome any inertia you may be feeling.

As with previous exercises, you may like to put the instructions on tape, or ask a friend or partner to talk you through it. You need to set aside at least half an hour of uninterrupted time.

First draw yourself an imaginary line on the floor and designate one end as the past and the other as the future (Figure 12.1). Step onto the line at the point that represents today **(1)**. Then ask yourself the following question.

- *What feelings am I experiencing today in connection with my career?* It may be anxiety, confusion, guilt, pressure, uncertainty. Or it may be excitement, anticipation, determination, purposefulness.

Once you have the feeling, ask yourself the following questions.

- *What is the reason for feeling this way?* It might be because something has happened to precipitate a move or change in your work. Or it might be

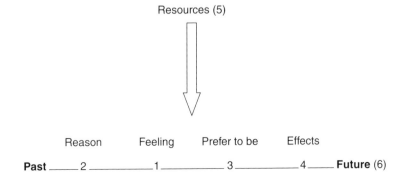

Figure 12.1

a bad experience, conflicting priorities, or because there is something you would like to do but someone has told you that you aren't up to it. Look to the past **(2)** to find out what it is, and place the reason on your imaginary line.

- *Where would you prefer to be, and when?* Given your current situation, what would you like instead? You may want to be in a new job, or to have started a course, or to have made an important decision. You may simply want peace of mind. When you think you know what it is you would like, ask yourself: 'If I had this thing, would I be happy?'. If you notice any doubts arising, adjust your goal until you are happy with it.

Once you have decided on what you would like, choose a point in the future when you would like it to be a reality. This may be a few weeks, six months or a year. One of the characteristics of people suffering from confusion and lack of direction in their careers is a great sense of urgency to sort it all out. Career development is not something to be rushed, however, so give yourself a comfortable deadline for your outcome if at all possible. Alternatively, if your goal is so ambitious that you are looking at more than a year before achieving it, try setting yourself an interim outcome.

Once you know when you would like to have achieved your goal, move along your line towards the future, to the point when you have achieved it **(3)**. This should be a pleasant place to be. Take a bit of time to feel the relief and pleasure of arriving there. What is it like? What are you feeling, seeing, hearing? What exactly have you achieved? What are your current circumstances? What is good about achieving this goal, and what difference does it make to your life?

- *What are the longer-term effects of having achieved your outcome?* Now imagine a time one or two years hence, a time when your career development process has really begun to bear fruit **(4)**. What are the effects of having achieved your outcome? What are you doing in your working life? Where are you and who is around you? What type of work are you doing and how are you enjoying it? What sort of income are you on and what effect is that having on your lifestyle? What are your hours and travel and benefits like? How is your personal life faring, and how are your family and friends responding to your new circumstances? How does all this make you feel?

Once you are thoroughly experiencing the pleasure of being in work you enjoy and value, take a look at the path behind you, and at the you of today and ask yourself the following question.

- *What did I do to reach where I am today? What resources did I use?* **(5)** The term 'resource' should be interpreted in the widest possible sense, and may include people, information services, reference libraries, books, websites, prospectuses, work experience, training opportunities, work experience and sources of funding. It will also include your personal resources, your strengths and skills, your experience and knowledge, your personal contacts, friends and supporters. Make a list of all these resources.

Now take yourself another five years into the future, and imagine what your life will be like then? (6) You have had five more years of enjoying the benefits of achieving your outcomes – where are you now and how does it feel? How are you feeling about yourself? About life in general? How is your personal life benefiting?

Finally, take yourself even further into the future, and imagine yourself at 80 years old. A wise, successful and experienced person who has enjoyed the benefits of personal fulfilment and job satisfaction for many years, look back on your career and recall your achievements, the challenges you have successfully faced, the mistakes you have learnt from and the benefits you have enjoyed. Take some time to fully experience the pleasure. When you are basking in this feeling of achievement and peace, look back at the you of today, standing there at point 5, and ask yourself the following question.

● *What personal resources, advice and beliefs would help the me of today?* Using the wisdom that has come from many years of experience, imagine you were able to give the you of today a bunch of balloons containing these resources and tips. What would they be? It may be confidence, a sense of perspective, motivation, courage, a knowledge that everything will be alright, calmness, a sense of purpose, a sense of fun or adventure, an appreciation of what you already have in your life, a knowledge that it is all a game, or a sense of humour. You may want to give yourself some advice on what to do, and how to do it, such as 'leave that job' or 'apply for that job' or 'ignore that person' or, more emphatically, 'just do it!', whatever 'it' might be.

When you have a full bunch of resource balloons, imagine sending them down to the you of today as a gift, and imagine the you of today accepting them gratefully, internalising them and basking in them. Take time for this to happen.

When you've done this, walk back along the line to the you of today and take a few moments to imagine yourself now with all those resources and knowledge of the future. What is different? What do you now know that you did not know before? What needs to be done? And most important of all, is the future sufficiently appealing for you to take the first steps towards it?

13

The three essential ingredients of career exploration

This chapter helps you to clarify what you need to do in terms of researching your options. By the end you should understand the importance and methods of:

- gathering information
- networking
- work experience.

If you decided that you wanted to buy an important piece of equipment, for example a stereo music system for your home, you would probably want to do some careful research. After all, we're talking significant money here. You would probably start off with some thoughts of what you want – is it for compact discs, cassettes, mini-discs, vinyl? Do you want it to be portable? How much power do you want from it? What is your budget? You would then want to look at what was available. You might ask around your friends, look in shops, catalogues and on websites. During this process you will gather some general information about each system's specifications and price, and begin to form a clearer idea of what you want. At this stage you will probably be able to whittle down your options to a handful, and then you might want to look more closely at these. You may go to the shop and have a listen, look in more detail at the features, compare prices. Once you have chosen a particular model, you may want to shop around for the best deal.

One more thing that most of us do, either consciously or subconsciously, is imagine what it would be like to have our machine. Perhaps we imagine lying on the sofa, lights dimmed, listening to our favourite CD. We may picture ourselves showing it off to our friends. Or we may envisage the pleasure of setting it all up, exploring the gadgets, and the satisfaction of getting it to work.

If you do go through these processes, the chances are that you will end up with a piece of equipment you are happy with. This isn't guaranteed, of course – you may be sold a faulty machine, or you may find that on further acquaintance there are aspects of the machine that you don't like, or hitherto unthought of requirements it does not fulfil. Nevertheless, you have substantially increased your chances of satisfaction.

While you would have thought that people would plan something as important as their career much more carefully than they would buying a piece of equipment, a surprising number of people take rather less trouble, resorting instead to methods such as:

- eliminating careers or work areas because of a bad experience in a particular job – this may have simply been due to an unpleasant colleague or boss
- extrapolating from good experiences – this may be just as risky as the former, e.g. if you work for a charismatic boss and mistake him or her for the work
- falling into careers by chance, applying for jobs because you happen to be there when they pop up and it seems like a good idea at the time
- taking advice from well-meaning onlookers. You meet up with someone who has just started a new job and they convince you that you would enjoy it too
- following parental wishes – that old but powerful chestnut.

These are all high-risk strategies, but if you've worked through this book then you are already a long way down the path to good career planning. You have looked at what you want from your career, explored what is available, and started to whittle down those options to a few that would fulfil your desires. You've also experienced what the future might bring by walking down that time line. The next stage is exploration, and the three essential areas of exploration in good career development are gathering information, networking and experience.

The ease and willingness with which you go through these processes will be dictated in part by your psychological type, so this is a good time to remind yourself of your preferences.

Gathering information

Critical for good decision making, information gathering can be done by talking directly to people (extroversion), reading (introversion), collecting facts (sensing) and exploring possibilities (intuition). You may obtain it through structured approaches (judging), or by taking in information as it arrives (perceiving). Whatever your preferences are, it is important to consider all these approaches, and to be aware of the methods you find less easy.

Accessing information in the modern world is becoming easier and easier, and the problem is more likely to be finding too much, rather than too little information. The Internet has revolutionised career research. Here you can find information on training and education, professional organisations, personal development, individual careers, commercial organisations, government departments, libraries, books, careers advisors and coaches, audiotapes, distance learning. Libraries are also an excellent source of a wide range of information, and many will have specialist careers advisors.

In the motivation exercise in Chapter 12, you gave some thought to the resources you could access. Review your list and see if there are any other sources of information you could use. Personal contacts are an excellent source of information, and these people may in turn be able to refer you to other people and other sources of information. Make a comprehensive list of every single source of information you can think of.

Networking

Personal contacts are crucial to good career planning. People are useful sources of information, as mentioned already, but they provide much more than factual help – they may have first-hand experience of particular jobs or careers, they will know other people in the same field, they will have heard of relevant organisations that you might not think to search for, they may even have courses or jobs on offer. They are excellent for filling in the gaps in the information you have already gathered, the detail, the more personal aspects of jobs or careers, the things that can't be found in formal sources. Meeting people also gives you the chance to assess the source of a piece of information or set of views. You may read a section in a careers book which raves about a particular career. This will have been written by an individual with a certain set of characteristics, experiences and views. These are bound to translate into personal agendas, tastes and prejudices. If you take these at face value you do so at your peril. Sitting down with someone enables you to see what they are like, and in particular to see if they are like you.

Another great advantage of networking is that it allows people to see you. Exposure is all when it comes to getting on in the world. You only have to look at the kinds of people who manage to achieve celebrity status to know that success has little to do with talent and everything to do with self-publicity. There is a great deal of difference between gradually increasing your circle of contacts and being on the front page of a national newspaper, but they are part of the same spectrum. Once you start on a programme of putting yourself about, it is truly amazing how quickly the number of people you know can multiply. When you meet someone new and they say, 'Ah, so you're Dick Jones', you know you're winning.

This part of the process tends to come more easily to those who prefer extroversion, who will often have many contacts already. But by no means all extroverts are happy to make cold contacts, and they do need to beware of talking too much at these encounters and so limiting their usefulness. These meetings should be predominantly fact-gathering, not fact-giving, missions, and while it is all too easy to talk about yourself and your career, the danger is that you come out with nothing of use.

Introverts, on the other hand, may need to force themselves to make contacts and are in danger of not making enough. Many years ago I went to see a careers counsellor and I can remember coming out in a cold sweat as she described to me the process of ringing people you didn't know, and giving false pretexts in order to ask disingenuous questions about the organisation they worked for. The combination of my preferences for introversion and feeling made this a totally unthinkable scenario, and while I learnt the power and importance of networking by forcing myself to make contacts, I did have to find methods with which I felt at least a modicum of comfort. People who prefer introversion may find networking difficult, but more positively they tend to be more concise and receptive in conversation, increasing the value of each encounter.

The secret for all types is to start with the contacts you have. Even if you can't think of anyone you know directly who can help you, ask your friends for contacts and you will be amazed at how many resources you have at your disposal before you make a single cold contact. Every time you talk to someone, ask 'Who else do you think it would be good to talk to?' If they can give you a personal introduction, so much the better. Often people are reluctant to make contacts, worrying that people are too busy or important to want to talk to little old them, but the truth is that most people love to be asked for help, especially when it is so easy for them to provide it. And they can always say 'no'.

Conferences and meetings are good places to make informal contacts. If you have a chance to go to a meeting where there are likely to be useful people for you to talk to, check if there is a delegate list and make a list of the people you want to approach. If you are not a natural mixer it is tempting to gravitate to the people you know at these events, so you may have to force yourself to walk across the room and introduce yourself to a stranger. Once you've done it a few times it becomes easier, partly because you have a few experiences under your belt which you have miraculously survived, but also because you start to accrue the benefits.

Tips for making the best of contacts

Plan your outcome

If you are planning a contact your first task is to decide what you want from it. This may sound a little mercenary, but you are on a quest here, and the best way to achieve any objective is to be clear what it is you are after. Also, if it is a busy person you are meeting, they will appreciate an early indication of what you want.

You may be after information, in which case be clear beforehand what exactly you are hoping to glean from the conversation. You may be after other contacts. If you are considering applying for a job in their organisation, you may simply want to find out what they are like, or what their organisation is like. You may want information or an opinion on someone else, something that needs to be handled with great caution and diplomacy. Whatever it is, be clear in your mind what you would like to have at the end of your conversation. Write it down if necessary, and prepare some questions.

Be interested

Every single person has one topic they find more interesting than anything else, and that is themselves. If you want to make a good impression on someone, or to get their co-operation, then show a genuine interest in them. If you want to talk to them then obviously you are interested in them, so this shouldn't be too difficult. If you can add to that some indication that you are impressed with them, they will be eating out of your hand in no time. There is no one whose opinion we value more than someone who thinks we're great. What great taste they have! Such good judgement!

The corollary of this is, beware of the temptation to talk about yourself. You may think that the whole point of making a contact is to run a personal advertisement, but if you want to annoy a busy person, this is an excellent way to do it. Once you have established rapport with the other person, you may want to drop in a couple of pieces of information about yourself to indicate what you have in common or what you may have to offer, but that's all. If you come out of an encounter having imparted more information than you have gained, then you need to review your technique.

Be prepared for rejection

If you follow these tips most of your experiences will be positive and you will be well on your way to becoming one of those people who, only months before, used to appall you with their shameless networking. From time to time, though, there are going to be people who don't want to talk to you, who aren't remotely interested in you and who clearly have much larger fish to fry. You may have found them on a bad day or at a bad time, in which case you could try approaching them on another occasion. They may have their own networking agenda and you are interrupting them. Or they may be one of those rare people who take more pleasure in making people feel small than they do in helping. It's helpful to remember that these people invariably have feelings of inadequacy which they try to overcome by feigning superiority. Whatever the reason, the important thing is not to take any of these rejections personally. Simply accept that it is going to happen from time to time, and move on.

Make networking a habit

Although networking is especially important when you are searching for career direction and jobs, it helps in all areas and at all stages of life. Networking within a workplace enables you to keep an eye on what is going on politically and socially, it gives you access to people who have skills and resources, it establishes a foundation for relationships that may prove valuable in the future. Networking at home supplies neighbours who will look after the cat when you're away, parents who will collect your children from school when you've been held up in a meeting, names of local traders for those plumbing and electrical disasters. Make networking a habit and you will be eternally thankful that you have.

Work experience

A young doctor came to see me. A few years before she had set out to specialise in thoracic medicine, but her training had been interrupted by a long period of illness. While she was now fit to return to work, she no longer felt equal to the unsociable hours, high pressure and long training involved in hospital medicine, and was contemplating general practice. It is a widely held misconception in the UK that general practice is an easy option. I asked her if she had ever spent any time in general practice. The answer was negative.

It is easy to gasp in astonishment at the notion that someone would plan to enter an area of work, perhaps for the rest of their working life, with no first-hand experience of that work. But it would be disingenuous to do so, for that is exactly what most people do.

Work experience can range from spending a few hours shadowing some-one who is doing the job, to doing the job for real for a while. What you choose will obviously depend on the opportunities available to you, and other practicalities such as time, finances and geography. It will also depend on how long you anticipate it taking to acquire sufficient flavour of the work and the environment to make an informed decision. Work experience is something you would usually arrange when you've done your research and made your contacts, and you need to bear it in mind as you go on your rounds.

In planning your experience you need to consider spending time in more than one place. Every workplace is individual in terms of the people, the environment and the work. Making a decision on the basis of a single experience exposes you to the same risks as mentioned above – an over-dependence on personalities and chance.

Work experience is an excellent opportunity to examine the content of a job in terms of your personal preferences, so do go armed with a good understanding of your preferences (*see* Chapter 6, p. 66) and your eyes open in terms of whether the work entails a predominance of:

- people and action; or time for reflection and working alone (E/I)
- attention to detail and practicalities; or complexity, abstraction and strategy (S/N)
- logical decision making and analysis; or understanding people and their needs (T/F)
- scheduled days with predictable deadlines; or flexible 'anything might happen' days.

As you would listen to a stereo system or test drive a car before you bought it, so too should you try out the careers or jobs you have in mind before committing yourself to them. Not only does it help you to decide if the career is for you, it looks excellent on your curriculum vitae and makes a good impression at interviews.

14

Action!

This chapter is designed to turn your knowledge, your options and your motivation into planned action. By the end you should:

- understand the principles of goal setting, and how type affects your approach
- have a set of written, validated goals
- know how to deal with common pitfalls
- have a system of time management for ensuring that your goals are achieved.

Few people will be strangers to the notion of 'to do' lists. We scribble down those tasks we need to do on scraps of paper, and they lie there, winking at us every time we sit at our desks or check the notice board. We have bursts of energy when we rush through a few, acting on those that have become crucial, indulging in the satisfaction of crossing them off, and every now and then taking the plunge with one of the less appealing items. Once a list has been around for a while, a few of the jobs have been ticked off and the piece of paper has begun to resemble a Jackson Pollock painting, most of us will run through it and transfer the outstanding tasks to a new piece of paper. Often those tasks are the same ones, week after week, and some jobs may stay on your list not only for months, but for years. You may even look at those items sometimes and ask yourself, how long will it take before I know I'm not going to do this?

The idea of this chapter is to learn how to turn a 'to do' list into an action plan; how to ensure that what goes on the list is realistic and is ticked off within a planned interval. It helps you to prioritise the demands on your time such that the important tasks get done and are no longer casualties of either trivia or crises.

The magic of goal setting

Many years ago I was working in a job I found thoroughly unsatisfying. The work itself was fine, but the climate of the organisation was controlling and petty, and while criticism flowed freely, appreciation was thin on the ground. I was dispirited. I had a colleague in the same department who was similarly disenchanted and the two of us developed a habit of going straight from work to her flat, where we achieved a certain catharsis in bemoaning our lot. There was a self-indulgent pleasure to be derived from moaning, and we certainly indulged.

As time went on, though, the pleasure faded and I began to feel not only disenchanted with work, but disenchanted with myself. I noticed that while my family and friends had been supportive and sympathetic for many months, of late their willingness to listen had ebbed somewhat. The still friendly but somewhat resigned looks on their faces were sufficient mirror for me to have a good view of myself. It was not an encouraging sight.

I decided to seek some professional help, and my first course of action was to send off for a career review pack. I waited for it to arrive with some excitement – there are few things more pleasurable than the feeling of taking charge after an extended period in 'victim' mode. When the parcel finally tumbled through my letterbox I was intrigued to find that included in the pack was an audio cassette labelled 'An excerpt from *The Psychology of Achievement*, by Brian Tracy'. With no idea of what to expect, I listened to it in my car as I travelled to and from work each day. It was interesting, very interesting. It covered all manner of intriguing and challenging ideas, such as the power of expectations and beliefs, the idea that we can achieve anything we want, and the relative unimportance of individual intelligence or ability as contributors to success. By far the most galvanising part, though, was the section on goal setting, and to this day I can hear Brian Tracy's voice as he intoned these profound words of warning:

'People who don't set goals are doomed forever to work for those who do.'

These words held an extraordinary power for me, for they opened up the possibility that there were two kinds of people in this world: a small number who are party to a secret which endows them with a magical ability to do whatever they want, and a much larger number, of whom I was clearly one, whose lives were destined to have all the direction of driftwood, tossed around as they were bound to be, by the ocean tides of the first group. This was a deeply unappealing picture, and while Tracy's claims of the almost mystical power of goal setting sounded a little far-fetched to my sceptical ears, this was surely something worth trying.

I put it to my friend, who, strangely enough, had also been moved to delve into the world of self-help and had come to similar conclusions. So it was that one dark winter's day the two of us retreated to the warm comfort of my friend's flat, not on this occasion with the intention of moaning, but with the intention of setting goals. Armed with only a pencil and paper, about two hours passed, following which we were both in possession of a single sheet of goals. On each piece of paper was written the overarching goal of finding a new job within a year. Interim goals included researching options, making contacts, exploring courses; everything we needed to do to move forward, and all with dates beside them. The tape instructed us to review our goals regularly, so we planned to meet monthly to review progress and set new goals.

Well, the weeks went by, the months went by and we didn't meet. Work pressures, home pressures, other priorities – we've all been there. After around six months, I remorsefully remembered my goals, the detail of which had been consigned to the unreachable parts of my brain, the physical evidence of which had disappeared into the profusion of paper in my office. I searched and searched, until at last I found them. I read through them: my short-term goals, my medium-term goals, and in total disbelief, I found I had achieved every single one. I was even on the point of achieving my overarching goal of finding a new job. It was uncanny, as if a hidden hand had been working behind the scenes. I was intrigued to see how my friend was getting on, and I found that she too had recently made the discovery that all her goals had mysteriously been met, without her consciously enacting them.

While there was no question that many of the items on our lists had been accomplished because we had personally taken action, the extraordinary part was that it had required no 'to do' list, no transferring of untackled tasks from one scrap of paper to another, no scheduling, no rushing and, perhaps above all, no effort. And there was something else that was strange. In among the tasks completed, the contacts made, the information gathered, were inexplicable coincidences – bumping into people who had just the piece of information we needed, or knew exactly the right person to talk to; stumbling over advertisements for courses or conferences that coincided precisely with our needs; encountering old friends whose lives were taking them down similar pathways and whose experiences we could learn from. The sum of all this, our actions and our synchronicities, was that we had both moved a very large step forward from where we had been on that winter's afternoon six months ago.

This experience gave us a very powerful message: not only could we make quite profound changes if we wanted to, but simply deciding to do so was enough. I was sufficiently moved and excited by this revelation to want to hand it on to someone, and that someone turned out to be my daughter. My daughter was then seven or eight years old, and because of the vagaries of the educational system with regard to birth dates, she had always been one of the youngest in her class at school. While a few months difference in age means little or nothing in older age groups, there is a world of difference between a child who is nearly five years old and one who is just four, and my daughter's relative youth had meant she had always had to work hard to keep up. Although these differences were beginning to fade by the time she was eight, and school was becoming easier for her, she was left with the erroneous belief that she wasn't any great shakes academically.

We had a chat one day in the school holidays and I asked her what she would like to achieve the following term. She told me she would like to do better in maths. I asked her how much better. She thought about it for a few moments, and then she said, 'I'd like to be top of the class'. I was quite surprised at the magnitude of this ambition, but I did my best to hide it, and asked her what she thought she would have to do to be top. She said she would need to concentrate in class, always ask the teacher if she didn't understand something and do some extra maths at home. I offered to help with the extra maths and asked her how much extra work she wanted to do. We settled on one session a week. And that's what we did. Just an hour or so every weekend, we sat down together and did some maths. By the end of term she was top of the class.

Since then, although I have regularly experienced the extraordinary power of goal setting, both personally and with clients, I have never ceased to be amazed by it.

The essentials of goal setting

Setting goals is the most powerful thing you will ever do in terms of achieving the working life you want, and if you apply it to other parts of your life, you will reap the rewards there too. There are a number of reasons why goal setting is so effective. First, it requires an explicit statement of what it is you want, and once you know where you want to go, you inexorably start moving in that direction. Second, setting goals requires a process of understanding what needs to be done to achieve your overall goal, and this again will inevitably move you in the right direction. Third, goal setting breaks down a large and possibly daunting ambition into a number of small, manageable steps. One of the main deterrents to career planning, especially if a major change is anticipated, is that it can be quite terrifying. Goal setting allows you to identify that ambition and then park it in a safe place while you consider much more approachable intermediate steps. Setting out to achieve a huge goal is like planning to swim the Atlantic before you can swim. It is fine to have an ambitious goal, but you need to set smaller interim goals if you are to have any hope of reaching it.

A goal is a specific measurable process or result you want to achieve within a particular time frame. Goals should always be stated in the positive, and they should begin with a verb. The problem with many New Year resolutions is that they are neither specific nor positive, and as a result they quickly fall by the wayside. Consider the example of someone who decides on the first of January that they are going to lose weight. This goal focuses on a negative, which is to weigh less. For a goal to be motivating, it has to be positive. Another flaw with this goal is that the statement is non-specific. On the one hand, the person can let themselves off the hook after losing the first couple of pounds. On the other, they neither know what it is they want, nor will they ever have the satisfaction of meeting a specific target.

Alternatives to this goal might be:

- to weigh x pounds by the end of March (a result)
- to eat 1000 calories a day for the next two months (a process)
- to fit into a specific item of clothing by April (a result)
- to walk three miles three times a week (a process).

The overarching goal may be to look in the mirror in six months' time and feel satisfied with what they see, but while this may act as a motivating vision of the future, in between there have to be some smaller, specific and realistic steps.

Notice the difference between specific and non-specific goals.

Specific and non-specific goals

Non-specific goal	*Specific goal*
Take more care of my health	Go to aerobics class twice a week
Reduce my stress level	Meditate at least 10 minutes every morning
Sort out my career	Write a career development plan
Explore a career option	See so and so next week
	Go to the library on Monday
	Look for courses on the Internet tonight

Goal setting and type

Goal setting is essentially a sophisticated form of list writing, so people who like to be scheduled and organised (judging) find that goal setting comes easily, and probably do some form of action planning already. However, they need to ensure that their planning does not preclude the possibility of following new directions if opportunities arise. The nature of career exploration is that it throws up many more possibilities than answers in the early stages. This can be unsettling for all types, but especially for judging types.

People who are flexible and like to keep their options open (perceiving) are good at adapting to changing circumstances and new opportunities, but may find goal setting harder as there are always new pathways appearing that look more attractive than the old ones. The danger here is that their flexibility may result in so many diversions that the essential tasks are never completed.

Similarly, intuitive and sensing types bring different strengths and weaknesses to the process. Intuitives are marvellous at looking ahead, imagining new possibilities and looking at the big picture. They can be lamentable at examining detail and practicalities. Sensing people find looking to the future a strain, and sometimes alarming, but when it comes to assessing the reality of a specific option, they are unsurpassable. Thinking types will find it easy to work out the pros and cons of a job at a safe distance, but may find this a limited tool for knowing how they will feel when actually doing a job. Feeling types are in danger of going for the 'feel' of a job and ignoring the logical reasons for and against.

All types need to be aware of their strengths and weaknesses, and to build on their strengths while working on their weaknesses. A good decision uses all four of the main functions (*see* Box below), and if you feel especially challenged by one or more of these, you might consider asking for assistance from someone with preferences that differ from your own.

Stages in good decision making

1   Assess the current situation, detail and practicalities (sensing)
2   Generate options (intuition)
3   Assess advantages and disadvantages of each option (thinking)
4   Assess effects on people involved, self and others (feeling)

Setting goals for career development

To set your goals, follow these steps.

1   *Write down your overarching goal for your career during the next period of your life.* The period may be six months or six years, and your goal may be to become a world expert on managing the incontinent patient, or simply to have clarity about what you would like to do next.
2   Consider what you will need to do to reach your overarching goal:
    – look at your list of career options, and sources of information and advice
    – consider any other actions you need to take to achieve your goal.
3   Set your goals under the following headings:
    – short-term goals (1–4 weeks)
    – medium-term goals (2–12 weeks)
    – longer-term goals (3–6 months)
    and write the date you will achieve it alongside each goal.
4   When you've finished, go through all your goals and check:
    – are they specific, measurable and with a time frame?
    – do they start with a verb?
    – are they either process or results-oriented, and do they contribute to the overarching goal?

Ensuring you achieve your goals

You have already taken the most important steps towards achieving your overall goal. The only obstacles to your progress now are:

● faults in the process so far
● falling into unexpected traps
● failing to make the time to achieve your goals.

To check for any faults in the process so far, you need to do a reality check. Look at your list of goals and ask yourself, 'Am I really going to do these things?' Whether or not you are going to do something will depend on the answers to the following questions.

● *Do your goals match your values?* If a goal is not in harmony with your values, the chances are you won't achieve it. Check each goal you have set against your personal values. What will achieving this goal get for you? What value will it satisfy? Sometimes we set goals that are more to do with proving ourselves than to do with what is important to us.

An individual might set a goal of achieving a certain income, or buying a particular car. The question is, what will that bring precisely? Similarly, a person might set their sights on a particular job, or level of seniority, but unless they are clear about what value that will satisfy, then they are unlikely to achieve it, and even if they do, they are unlikely to feel satisfied. If you find a goal that is more to do with external appearances than internal values, then chuck it out. It will divert your energies from what really matters to you, and the rewards will be few.

Your goals must also consist of desires, not 'shoulds'. People's ambitions are full of 'shoulds'. The danger of these is that when you achieve them they fail to deliver in terms of satisfaction or fulfilment. Success has been described as 'achieving something you thought you wanted 20 years ago'. Delete any 'shoulds' from your list.

- *Are you willing to be responsible for your goals?* Ask yourself if you are willing to take responsibility for the goals you have set, or are you half hoping someone else will make them happen for you? If you are not willing to take responsibility for them, out they go.
- *Are the benefits sufficiently motivating?* Take yourself into the future and imagine having achieved your goals. How does it feel? Is it good enough to motivate you to carry out your goals?
- *Are you prepared for any negative consequences?* Finally, check if there are any down sides to achieving any of your goals. Will anyone object? Are there likely to be any side effects? If so, are you prepared for these consequences? If not, you can be sure you won't do them.

As you do these checks you may find you need to make some adjustments. If you really can't see yourself achieving one or more of your goals, there may be interim steps you need to take, or maybe another approach is needed. Again, if any of your goals conflict with your values, you may need to rethink those goals; and if imagining achieving all your goals does not fill you with happiness and energy, perhaps you are not aiming high enough; perhaps you need a new and more exciting overall goal. Setting goals is all about creating a game you can win. Make it easy and enjoyable for yourself.

Common pitfalls

Fear

This is the one thing that is most likely to stop you achieving your goals. Fear is dependent on negative thoughts. It is produced when instead of thinking about what it will be like when you have achieved your goals, you are thinking about what it will be like when you fall at the first hurdle. If you picture your mind as an open birdcage, and your thoughts as birds, there is little you can do to stop the birds flying in. Your choice is in what you do with them once they're there. You can feed them and feed them so they become fatter and unable to fly out again, or you can simply open the door on the other side and let them fly out.

Another way of combating fear is not to look too far ahead or behind, but to focus on your current goals. Anyone with a fear of heights will tell you that the only way to contain fear when ascending a ladder, for example, is to not look up, *definitely* not look down, but to focus on each step as you take it.

Negativity from other people

Be prepared to find that people around you do not share your enthusiasm for your plans. Change and purpose in others can be unsettling, and it is important to remember that people's negativity almost always comes from what your plans make them feel about *themselves* and their lives. It does not come, as is often presented, from an objective view about the sanity of your proposals. There is great comfort in stability and being the same as others – that is, after all, why it takes us so long to make changes. Seeing someone else making changes while we remain the same, can give feelings of discomfort and of being 'left behind'. Partners, in particular, may wonder if the new exciting you is still going to find them interesting.

Pushing too hard

It can be tempting to think that if you try till it hurts it will all be worth it in the end. That is no way to have a nice life. In the game of bagatelle, you fire a ball into play and you wait till it falls. You then retract the spring and wait for another ball to appear before you fire it. You don't keep retracting the spring and firing at air. That would be tiring and unproductive. Action is good, but so is waiting for things to come to you. If you are not enjoying the process you are pushing too hard. Finding the right career pathway takes time, and rushing the process only increases the risk that you leave important stones unturned in the quest for a quick solution.

The 'I don't have time' demon

This is possibly the most invidious of all pitfalls, and deserves special attention.

How to manage your time effectively

If you can manage your time well, you are on the way not only to career success, but success in every sphere of your life. There is a popular story that illustrates perfectly the difference that skills in this area can make to what you manage to achieve in your day-to-day life.

A professor was teaching a group of students. On the table was a large glass jar, a number of rocks, a bowl of sand and a jug of water.

The professor selected a student. 'Please fill the glass jar with rocks,' the professor said. The student did so. 'Is the jar quite full?', the professor asked the students. The students agreed it was.

'Now, pour the sand into the jar until it reaches the top.' The student did so. Again the professor asked if it was full, and the students agreed it was.

Then, the professor said, 'Now pour the water in'. The student did so, until the water brimmed over the top.

What we tend to do in our busy lives is to pour the water in first. We then attempt to pour in the sand, and the ensuing mess ensures that we don't even think about putting in the rocks. Putting in the rocks first ensures that the important stuff gets done, which is in itself a sufficient reward to energise you for the smaller, less important tasks. There are many different models of time management, but the following one, adapted from Stephen Covey's *Seven Habits of Highly Effective People*, is specifically geared to increasing the chances of the rocks finding their way into the jar (Figure 14.1).

Our activities may be grouped as either important or not important, and either urgent or not urgent. In the 'Important/Urgent' quadrant (quadrant 1) are the activities a working and domestic life are full of; the actions you take in response to other people and events. Consisting of letters, phone calls, meetings and crises, they also hold in their ranks those things that used not to be urgent, but having been transferred from list to list for some considerable time, have now become so. Important and urgent activities are energy consuming, may be stress inducing and they expand to fit the time available. If you allow them to, they will ensure you never reach any of your important but not urgent tasks, and will wear you out sufficiently to drive you into the 'Not urgent/Not important' quadrant, thus wasting time in unrewarding activities that you do because you don't have the energy to do anything else.

If you are someone with a preference for doing things in good time (judging) the 'Important/Urgent' quadrant causes particular difficulty. People

	Urgent (Reactive)	Not urgent (Elective)
	1	**2**
Important	Crises, responding to demands, some meetings, deadlines, answering calls	**Your goals**, planning, relationship building, values clarification, quality leisure and relaxation
	3	**4**
Not important	Some meetings, conversations, duties, phone calls	Time-wasting activities (you know what these are)

Figure 14.1

who prefer judging find it extremely difficult to do non-urgent tasks when they know there are urgent ones to be done. The result is that the non-urgent ones, which may be as simple and important as having fun, are never reached. Furthermore, judging types tend to find urgent tasks inherently unsatisfying, as they have to be done quickly, rather than in the scheduled and comfortable mode that is their preference.

Flexible, spontaneous people who prefer perceiving may find that tasks have to reach the 'Urgent/Important' quadrant in order to generate the impetus to tackle them. While perceiving types enjoy putting in last-minute effort, the problem with this is that some important activities may never become urgent and are therefore never tackled. Relationship building, for example, is only likely to become urgent when you need something from someone in a crisis. It is because you need to have a foundation for a relationship if you are going to tap its reserves in a crisis that it must be built at less-pressing times.

Many of the categories of activity to be found in quadrant 1 may also be found in the 'Urgent/Not important' quadrant 3, demands which appear urgent but do not really need to be done at all. In working life, meetings can often fall into this category. It is not always easy to tell if an activity is important, but if it doesn't feed into your values or goals in some way, then it probably isn't. A good way of finding out if an activity is important or not is to consider what would happen if you didn't do it. Better still, if somewhat risky, is to stop doing it and see what happens.

After I had given a seminar on time management once, a woman came up to me. She was doing a high-level job in a government department and had recently reduced her hours to three days a week in order to spend more time with her two young children. As is often the case, she had been allowed to reduce her hours, but her responsibilities had remained the same. The result was that every Monday she went to work, rested and happy from four days at home, and within about 15 minutes she was in a state of high anxiety. Her in-tray would be piled high, the telephone would ring incessantly, everybody wanted to see her and she had no time to do the important developmental work for her job – writing reports, starting new projects and keeping up with new technology. One day, she told me, she decided to see what happened if she didn't go through her in-tray. It took an inordinate amount of her time, and she had an idea that if she left it, most of it would look after itself. So she had a quiet and productive week or so, using the freed-up time to tackle long-neglected tasks. Everything was fine until about ten days into the experiment.

The first indication that all was not well was an irate person on the telephone, saying that he had missed a meeting because he hadn't been sent any papers. She then discovered she had a meeting scheduled for the next day, and her boss had written her a note the previous week asking her to fix the agenda. A politician wanted to know why no one had replied to his urgent request for information. She found she had missed a deadline for commenting on a crucial report. In short, the brown stuff hit the fan in spectacular fashion.

'It was awful' she laughed, 'but it did teach me a great deal. It made me realise, of course, that the time I spent going through my in-tray was in fact important. I also discovered that there were only a small number of things in my in-tray that needed to be dealt with urgently, and that they could be identified reasonably easily. So I sat down with my secretary and we developed a system where the post was divided into important and urgent, important but not urgent, and not important. That made life much more manageable.'

The rocks, of course, are to be found under 'Important/Not Urgent', in quadrant 2. They are the most important things in your life and will pay the greatest dividends if you do them. Because they are satisfying, they give you the energy you need to accomplish the mundane but necessary tasks in life. If you neglect them, one of two things will happen: either they eventually move into the 'Important/Urgent' quadrant, where they have the capacity to cause immense stress, or they drop off the list altogether.

Among the activities in quadrant 2 are, of course, your goals. If you are ever to have the life you want, it is essential that you schedule time for these. Also in this quadrant you will find relationships. It is all too easy to go into work with the idea that the tasks are the important part, and good relationships are a luxury that you indulge in when there is time. If you think this way, in even a moderately busy job, relationships are liable to fall way down the list of priorities, until such time as a 'hello' in the morning feels like all you can afford. The result is loss in every way, for other people are the key to effectiveness and peace of mind. If you haven't built relationships, how can you delegate effectively? How can you co-operate with others for maximum effect? How do you enlist people's help in a crisis?

Also in quadrant 2 you find fun and genuine leisure. Leisure time and holidays are not a luxury. They are essential for keeping the human machine in good nick, and need to be scheduled along with all the other activities in quadrant 2.

Leisure time and holidays are not a luxury.

It is possible to do all the necessary groundwork for your career, but unless the fruits of your work translate into action, you will remain stationary. Goal setting and the planned and effective use of your time will ensure that all your hard work results in a working life that provides satisfaction, fulfilment and happiness.

Things which matter most must never be at the mercy of things which matter least.
Goethe

15

The top ten tips for a happy and successful career

This book represents only the beginning of career development, but it is arguably the most important and most often neglected part. There are many books on applying for jobs, writing CVs and going for interviews, and the advice on these skills varies enormously from country to country, year to year and profession to profession. What is discussed in this book does not change. It can provide the foundation for anybody's life, wherever you are and whoever you are, teenager or pensioner, street sweeper or royalty, black or white, male or female, rich or poor. And it is likely to be as applicable to people's lives in 100 years' time as it is today.

I have a belief that the kind of groundwork that is covered in this book is a required course, and that we take each part of that course when the time is right. Most people looking back at their lives so far will find patterns in their experiences. These patterns represent the lessons that life is trying to teach us, guiding us towards what is ultimately right for us, and the hard truth is that the lessons will be repeated as often as it takes for us to learn them.

So career and personal development is a continuous process. At any point along the way it can be useful to revisit the kinds of thoughts and processes covered in this book. Our values change, we change, our attitudes to money and meaning change, our skills, experience and knowledge constantly grow, and there will always be more limiting beliefs to work on. Our fundamental personality type is something that is always with us, but it too develops over time. You tend to get better at using your favourite functions once you become aware of them. Later in life you learn to use your less preferred functions, and at any time you may want to give your dominant functions a rest. All this may lead to new interests and desires.

And, of course, we're all human, so we lapse. Our lives get out of balance again, we find ourselves doing things we don't value, and our list of goals becomes dog-eared and out of date. But emotions have a habit of telling us when we're off track, and at these times it helps to go back to first principles. If you do that regularly, you will gradually build a solid foundation of values and sense of purpose that both guides you towards happiness and fulfilment in your life and protects you when things go wrong.

Over the past ten years I have read no end of books on career and personal development, and what I have noticed is that the more I read, the less likely I am to find something entirely new. I have come to realise that there is a fount of wisdom out there that is as old as the hills, and that the job of each writer is to present it in a new and different way in the hope that it will reach a new and different audience. What I have attempted to do in these final pages is to pass on to you a small part of the collective wisdom that exists in relation to work.

The top ten tips

1   **If you keep moving towards what is important to you, the world will make it possible for you.** Once you've done the groundwork for your career there's a chance that the perfect working life you have conceived on the inside may fail to be mirrored in the form of a career or job on the outside. Given the uniqueness and complexity of each person, that is hardly surprising. But the strange thing is that once you know what it is you want, if you keep moving towards it in whatever way you can, the world miraculously moulds itself around your desires. Career development is about choosing, not once, not twice, but continually through your life, often in quite small ways. And if you choose repeatedly on the basis of your values, it is not probable, but inevitable, that you will find work that you love.

2   **The most satisfying kind of work is that which makes a contribution that you personally value.** You may be doing a great job of fitting limb prostheses, and as a result many millions of people may be able to do things they otherwise could not, but if you are more interested in people's minds than their bodies, you are unlikely to feel fulfilled. You may be an excellent occupational therapist or physiotherapist or nurse, helping many people a day to deal with their problems and live productive lives, but if your heart lies in using your practical skills to make beautiful furniture for people's homes, then you are unlikely to feel fulfilled.

It is when your gifts and values get together, and allow you to give something superb that you think is important, that you are likely to experience satisfaction and fulfilment. You may find that in the form of a single career, or you may find it in a myriad of small ways.

3   **Work is to be enjoyed, not endured.** If you plan your career in order to reach a specific destination as fast as possible, you are at risk of giving up enjoyment in the short to medium term in return for something you think you want in the long term. Then, if you don't achieve success in the way you have defined it for yourself, you are likely to feel disappointed and a failure. If you do succeed, the chances are high that you will also be disappointed, partly because success alone is rarely satisfying, and partly because you may get there only to find that you no longer want it.

It is the journey, not the destination that is important, and the journey is more likely to resemble a sailing trip than a beeline. A sailing boat has a general idea about where it wants to go, but only when the wind is directly behind can it head straight for its destination. More often it is travelling at an angle, enjoying the scenery en route.

Allowing for the fact that working life will not necessarily be easy all the time, if you are not enjoying yourself overall, you may be neglecting yourself. It may be because you are pushing too hard, instead of waiting for things to come to you. It may be that you have sacrificed too much in order to reach a particular place in your career. Or it may be that you are on the wrong track, living and working outside your values. Work should be enjoyable.

4   **Few decisions are bad decisions, and even fewer are irreversible.** Many a career crisis centres around 'either/or' decisions, and what turns a dilemma into a crisis is the belief that there is a right or wrong decision, and that if you make a 'wrong' decision it will be disastrous.

Realising that a decision between options is really a choice of different experiences, all of which are likely to be valuable, and that if you don't enjoy one experience you can always choose another, turns decision making into a completely different phenomenon. It is also helpful to realise that if you are choosing between two compelling options, the chances are that there exists a third, or even a fourth option that will bring you the best of both. And if you are having extreme difficulty deciding between several options, you probably have several excellent options on your hands, and the decision as to which one you go with may not be as important as you think.

5   **Your heart is your best guide.** Your inner guide, intuition, gut feeling, whatever you like to call it, is the best guide to what you are meant to be doing with your life. Your brain is very useful for many things, but it has a tendency to pour cold water on your dreams. Become aware of the 'fears, doubts and disillusions' radio station and turn it off.

6   **The world is a much bigger place than the one you currently occupy, and the boundaries you see are mostly imaginary.** Try

doing something completely new one day and you will find a different world, populated by people doing things you have hitherto been entirely unaware of. You could take a class in a subject you've never considered before; or go to a foreign country; or look at pictures in *National Geographic*; or do some voluntary work with people sleeping rough; or work in a charity shop; or help in a drug rehabilitation centre; or just talk to people in a bus queue. You may not be aiming at a completely different life, but just knowing it is there if you want it can be extraordinarily liberating.

7   **Life is not about what happens to you, it's about what you do in response.** Your control over what happens to you is moderate, your control over how you respond is potentially absolute. It's wonderful when life goes smoothly for a while, when you succeed, get along with people, earn money and achieve status. But life is not about everything going well, and neither is work. It is about becoming the person you want to be. All our experiences, good and apparently bad, are opportunities to move one step closer to being that person, to create ourselves anew. If everything went smoothly we would have the emotional and mental maturity of a toddler.

   When something unpleasant happens, the tendency is to dwell on its awfulness. Unless it is something you can change, much more useful is to ask yourself: 'Who do I want to be in relation to this?'

8   **Life is much more than a career.** Whatever is important to us in life, a career is just one of several places in which we may find it. To find work that is uplifting, enjoyable and allows you to contribute the very best you have to offer is wonderful, but pouring all your efforts into any one area of life inevitably means neglecting other areas. The consequence is not only a lack of balance in your life, but that when you lose your work, there is little to fall back on. Work is important, but it is not everything.

   A senior British politician, Michael Portillo, whose chances of becoming prime minister were blown by admitting his sexuality, had this to say on his retirement from politics:

   'I don't think I will merit more than a footnote in the history of the Conservative party. But along the way I discovered that life and career are not the same thing. Many people are miserable until they find that out.'
   Michael Portillo, *Sunday Times*, 22 February 2004

9   **Happiness comes from the inside, not the outside.** If you are always striving towards something in the belief that it will make you happy,

you will forever be disappointed. Observations of people who undergo either major success or major trauma in their lives have shown that both happiness and unhappiness in relation to external events is short-lived, and that people tend to return to their pre-event state in a matter of weeks. Happiness is a state of being, not a state of having, and being happy leads to success, not the other way round.

10   **The most effective thing you can do for your career is to look after yourself, your health and your spirits.** The saying that the greatest resource you have is yourself has been repeated so often it has become a cliché. Nevertheless it is true. There are people who work hard all the time. It may be in their career, or it may be looking after a family, or some other area of life. They feel a drive to give everything to that cause, and simply don't have time to care for themselves. But in the end something will always give. It may be mental or physical ill health, it may be burnout, it may be flagging performance or mistakes made through loss of perspective, or it may be divorce or loss of friends and family. Like any machine, human beings need regular care and maintenance, and lack of attention to these needs is likely to result in poor performance and early breakdown.

If happiness breeds success, it follows that if you want to be successful you need to get happy and stay happy. Getting and staying happy involves looking after yourself: finding people who support you, reading inspiring books and articles, taking holidays, exercising, relaxing, eating well, making friends, doing things you enjoy, paying attention to the people you love, and developing and educating yourself. Looking after yourself is not a luxury, but a prerequisite for wellbeing and success.

And finally . . .

The ideas and techniques in this book are tried and tested ways of helping people to get off the treadmill for a while and think, what is really important in my working life, and how can I ensure that it is full of those things? This may seem a rather self-centred approach, but the truth is that when people are happy, they bring that sense of well being to their work, their play and their relationships. When that happens, everyone benefits.

Bibliography

- Bloom W (2001) *The Endorphin Effect*. Piatkus.
- Boldt LG (1993) *Zen and the Art of Making a Living: a practical guide to creative career design*. Penguin.
- Charvet SR (1997) *Words That Change Minds*. Kendall/Hunt Publishing.
- Clarke J (2000) *The Money or Your Life*. Century (Random House Group).
- Covey SR (1990) *The 7 Habits of Highly Effective People*. Simon and Schuster.
- de Botton A (2000) *Consolations of Philosophy*. Hamish Hamilton.
- Ditzler J (1994) *Your Best Year Yet*. Thorsens.
- Goleman D (1996) *Emotional Intelligence*. Bloomsbury Publishing.
- Handy C (1998) *The Hungry Spirit*. Arrow Books.
- Harris T (1995) *I'm OK, You're OK*. Arrow Books.
- Jeffers S (1991) *Feel the Fear and Do It Anyway*. Arrow Books.
- Jung C (1933) *Modern Man in Search of a Soul*. Harcourt Brace Jovanovich.
- Owen N (2001) *The Magic of Metaphor*. Crown House Publishing.
- Tracy B. *The Psychology of Achievement*. Audio CDs.

Index